D0998408

DATE DUE

THE
FIGHT
TO
SURVIVE

THE
FIGHT
TO
SURVIVE

A YOUNG GIRL, DIABETES,
AND THE DISCOVERY OF INSULIN

CAROLINE COX

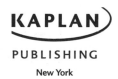

KAPLAN

PUBLISHING

New York

This publication is designed to provide accurate and authoritative information in regard to the subject matter covered. It is sold with the understanding that the publisher is not engaged in rendering legal, accounting, or other professional service. If legal advice or other expert assistance is required, the services of a competent professional should be sought.

Published by Kaplan Publishing, a division of Kaplan, Inc.
1 Liberty Plaza, 24th Floor
New York, NY 10006

Printed in the United States of America

10 9 8 7 6 5 4 3 2 1

Library of Congress Cataloging-in-Publication Data

Cox, Caroline, 1954–
    The fight to survive : a young girl, diabetes, and the discovery of insulin / Caroline Cox.
        p. ; cm.
    Includes bibliographical references and index.
    ISBN 978-1-60714-551-6
    1. Gossett, Elizabeth Hughes, 1908–1981—Health. 2. Diabetics—New York—Biography. 3. Diabetes—History. 4. Insulin—History. I. Title.
    [DNLM: 1. Gossett, Elizabeth Hughes, 1908-1981. 2. Diabetes Mellitus, Type 1—United States—Biography. 3. Diabetes Mellitus, Type 1—history—United States. 4. Drug Discovery—history—United States. 5. History, 20th Century—United States. 6. Insulin—history—United States. WZ 100 C8773f 2009]
    RC660.4.C695 2009
    618.92′462—dc22

                                                                        2009019112

Kaplan Publishing books are available at special quantity discounts to use for sales promotions, employee premiums, or educational purposes. For more information or to purchase books, please call the Simon & Schuster special sales department at 866-506-1949.

To the memory of my father,

William (Bill) Thomson,

1924–1978

CONTENTS

PROLOGUE

IN JULY 1922, 14-YEAR-OLD Elizabeth Evans Hughes lay near death. At slightly under five feet tall, she weighed only 45 pounds, less than half the normal weight for a girl her height. She was emaciated, and her abdomen and pelvic bones were protruding. Her skin was dry and scaly, her hair was thin, and her muscles were wasted. She felt so weak that she could barely stand up, and walking was difficult.

Her parents watched her carefully, alert for signs of further deterioration in her condition that would signal the end. It was a grim duty. Her father at least had the relief of going out to work each day, although as the front door closed behind him, he could never be sure he would see Elizabeth alive when he returned. Her mother faced the daily struggle of watching helplessly as her daughter slipped away.

What had happened to this once healthy girl who enjoyed all the advantages of a stable, well-connected, loving family? Elizabeth's nightmare had begun in the fall of 1918, when she was 11 years old. One day, she had gone to a friend's birthday party and had especially enjoyed the chance to eat cake and ice cream, foods her mother did not usually let her eat. But when she came home she was thirsty—so thirsty that she drank quarts of water. As the weeks passed, she felt increasingly tired. When she went to other parties and had the opportunity to eat sweet treats, she felt so thirsty afterward that she was frantic if she could not quickly get water to drink. Her mother also noticed that her usually energetic daughter was often listless and needed to urinate a lot, but she still seemed to be eating heartily, and surely that was a good thing. Mrs. Hughes watched Elizabeth nervously, unsure of what was wrong. There had been a polio epidemic in the city only two years earlier and as winter approached, there was an alarming increase in the number of cases of influenza. She worried about both those possibilities. When Elizabeth came down with flu later that winter it seemed to explain everything, but when she recovered in early spring 1919, she was still often thirsty, was urinating more than usual, and was losing weight.

Her doctor suspected she had diabetes. He recommended that her parents take her to see Frederick Allen, one of the world's leading specialists in that illness. Allen confirmed the diagnosis. Elizabeth had what we now know as type 1, juvenile diabetes, or insulin-dependent diabetes mellitus. Today, IDDM is treatable with insulin and a controlled diet. In 1919, before the discovery of insulin, sufferers declined rapidly and then faced certain death.

Scientists of the time were close to understanding diabetes but not close to any long-term treatment. They knew that it caused the pancreas, a gland in the abdomen, to stop secreting a substance that regulated the way the body metabolized carbohydrate, but no one had yet been able to isolate and identify what that secretion was. Many of the top diabetes specialists and researchers, such as Allen and the Boston-based Elliott Joslin, were optimistic that a treatment or cure might be found in their lifetimes, but they held out little hope that it would be in time for any patients under their current care. As Allen considered Elizabeth's future, he calculated it in months.

Elizabeth's symptoms reflected the vicious cycle of the disease. She was hungry and ate well, but her body was not metabolizing food efficiently. She was losing weight because, unable to absorb new sources of food energy, her body was burning its stores of fat. She urinated a lot because the unmetabolized sugars in the body spilled into her urine, increasing its volume. Unable to absorb fluids efficiently, and losing them at an excessive rate, she was constantly thirsty.

Her weight loss, listlessness, hunger, and thirst were just the visible symptoms of her illness. Internally and unseen, it was beginning to do terrible damage. Without this unknown secretion from the pancreas, acids called ketones would clog her organs (a condition called keto-acidosis). Over time, her body would become unable to metabolize a range of other nutrients in addition to carbohydrate, and all this in turn would eventually lead to kidney failure. Ultimately, she would lose all appetite and sink into a coma. Death would follow a few hours later.

Elizabeth was not alone in her suffering, nor was her family alone in its grief. Many people suffered from the disease. Doctors were puzzled, because the illness seemed sometimes to be severe or acute and at other times mild. They were confused by the range of people affected—old and young, rich and poor, fat and thin, men and women. Today we know that they were looking at two different kinds of diabetes. In type 1 diabetes, more common in children and young adults, the pancreas fails to produce the secretion, which we now know to be the hormone insulin; and in type 2, more common in older adults and the obese, the body has become resistant to insulin and is not metabolizing the insulin it produces. In both types, the presence of sugar in the urine is the principal means of identifying the disease, which is why doctors thought they were looking at the same illness. The symptoms of type 2 diabetes are more subtle than those of type 1 and some people can have it for years without knowing, attributing their listlessness to other factors. At the beginning of the 20th century, both kinds of diabetes together affected perhaps as much as 2 percent of the U.S. population and millions more across the world. While acute (type 1) diabetes killed in months, "mild" (type 2) was equally fatal over the long term. Elliott Joslin's records show that no diabetic of any kind under his care survived more than ten years after diagnosis.

But Frederick Allen had recently developed a treatment plan that was Elizabeth's best hope for prolonging her life. The principle behind his diet was that patients should consume only as much food as their bodies could efficiently metabolize, however little that was. This treatment plan required beginning an extremely low-carbohydrate diet and raising it slowly to the point where sugar appeared in the urine. When that point was reached, one knew the limit of one's tolerance and could stay below it. Today for sufferers of type 2 diabetes, what Allen called mild diabetes, diet alone can sometimes allow people to lead a normal, healthy life. For type 1 or acute diabetics, such as Elizabeth, levels of tolerance are extremely low, and staying below them meant living on very little food. Early death was still inevitable, but if patients adhered to his strict diet they could prolong their lives and relieve the distress of the otherwise inevitable organ failure.

Allen's diet plan was known as "starvation therapy." For Elizabeth, it meant living on an average of about 800 or fewer calories a day instead of the 2,000 or so normal for a girl her age. Certainly, it would prevent the sugar in her body from reaching toxic levels. But, instead, she would slowly fall prey to a variety of infections to which she had no resistance. It was a sad irony that Elizabeth and other diabetics could prolong their lives only by starving themselves to death.

Not surprisingly, few people could endure the relentless hunger of such a diet. Some of Allen's patients agreed to be kept as virtual prisoners in his clinic to help them stay on it. Even then, some patients sneaked in extra food whenever possible. Few of those who lived at home could stick to the diet, and those who did were often overwhelmed by weakness and the misery of the daily regimen and rarely left their rooms.

Elizabeth was different. Living at home, she adhered diligently to her diet. It had a weekly cycle. For six days, she could eat her full allowance of about 800 calories. This was followed by a "half day" or "fast day," when she consumed about 400 calories before beginning the week anew. On the days she could eat the most, her meals, with small variations, consisted of a small bowl of oatmeal for breakfast, perhaps an egg for lunch, and a piece of chicken or a lamb chop for dinner with some vegetables cooked three times to remove the carbohydrate from them—along with any flavor.

For three years, she faced continuous hunger but stayed on Allen's plan. Certainly, others helped her do so. She was under the watchful eye of her nurse, Blanche Burgess, and occasionally her mother, but she was far from being a prisoner. Elizabeth's self-discipline and dogged determination kept her on her track.

Yet Elizabeth rejected the identity of an invalid. Diabetes and indeed many other chronic illnesses are isolating, but she refused to be physically or mentally confined. She read widely and wrote essays for competitions in children's magazines, the results of which she would not know for months. She took delight in music and went for walks, using up her small store of energy to enjoy nature. Most surprisingly, she continued to engage with the world around her, spending time with family friends at teas and dinners. On those occasions she was surrounded by food she could not eat, more nurtured by the company than she was tortured by the sight and smell of food. She tried her best in the face of enormous challenges to live well.

Elizabeth never lost hope that she was living a life that would continue, and so she invested in it and in her friends. She made the effort to stay part of communities of readers, birdwatchers, nature-lovers, opera buffs, and travelers. With these people, she was not the stoic diabetic. She was a girl who loved fast boats, who dreamed of riding in airplanes, and enjoyed any book about travel and adventure. She joked with her mother about when she might marry. When her parents forbade her to go up for a joyride in an airplane, she retorted that she would simply do it on her 21st birthday when she became a legal adult. When she became so weak that walking was a struggle, she decided she would be a writer when she grew up, because then it would not matter that she could not use her legs. She made plans for vacations for months and seasons ahead. She was claiming her life on her own terms.

But she was wasting away. Her parents watched powerless, their great social and financial resources of no use to them in this crisis. Charles and Antoinette Hughes were both well educated and socially elite. Antoinette Carter Hughes was the daughter of a prosperous New York lawyer who could trace her lineage back to the *Mayflower*. Charles Evans Hughes came from more humble origins but had had a meteoric rise to fame and modest fortune. After becoming a successful lawyer, he had been Republican governor of the state of New York. He was then appointed as a justice to the U.S. Supreme Court in 1910, only to step down from the position in the summer of 1916 to accept the Republican Party's nomination for the presidency. That November, he lost a heartbreakingly close presidential race to the incumbent, Woodrow Wilson. The family then returned to New York, where Hughes practiced law and argued cases in front of the Supreme Court on which he had once sat. As Elizabeth became frail, Hughes again entered public life and became secretary of state under President Warren Harding. He was now one of the most powerful men in the world—but was powerless to save his daughter's life.

In May 1922, a glimmer of hope appeared. As Hughes was being sworn in to office the previous year, a group of men had come together at the University of Toronto in Canada to commence a series of experiments to try to identify the elusive pancreatic extract. They were not the first to search for it and they hoped that, at least, their work would add to the growing body of knowledge about the way the pancreas worked. A year later, after many frustrations, they had made a major breakthrough: they identified an extract from animal pancreas and found a way of treating it so that it might help human diabetics. They called the extract insulin. In May, they presented their findings at a scientific conference and all the doctors and researchers present, including Frederick Allen, recognized it immediately as a great discovery. However, this was still in the early days. The drug could be made only in very small quantities, not nearly enough even to begin systematic human clinical trials.

The Hugheses eagerly read the newspaper reports and knew they needed to be patient. But by early summer, Elizabeth had experienced a catastrophic decline. Antoinette Hughes decided to contact Dr. Frederick Banting in Toronto, the researcher whose name she had seen mentioned in the press in connection with the discovery. She wrote to him in early July to see whether Elizabeth might be able to get some of the new drug. Her daughter, she wrote, was "pitifully depleted and reduced." Despite her pleas and her political clout, Banting could not help her. He sent her the same response he sent to the other desperate families who had contacted him since the news was released. He was sorry, but there was very little insulin available and he could not predict when there would be more. Antoinette Hughes resigned herself to watching her daughter die.

Elizabeth, meanwhile, had decided she would be her famous father's biographer. As her mother was writing to Banting in desperation, Elizabeth used her savings to buy herself a portable typewriter to prepare for her future career as a writer.

CHAPTER 1

The Dread Diabetes

THROUGH THE FALL of 1918 and the winter that followed, Charles and Antoinette Hughes had watched their energetic and sporty daughter grow pale and thin. Over those months, her weight dropped from 75 pounds, average at the time for a slender girl with her approximately four-foot-eleven inch frame, down to 65. She looked like a wraith. In March 1919, their local doctor made a preliminary diagnosis of diabetes. It filled the Hugheses with dread, and it was with heavy hearts that they took Elizabeth to the famous diabetes specialist Frederick Allen. Dr. Allen could do nothing to assuage their fears. As soon as he saw Elizabeth and heard her symptoms, he had no doubt as to the diagnosis. A test of her urine and blood confirmed it. He was equally certain of her fate: death.

It was no comfort to know that Elizabeth was dying from one of humanity's oldest known diseases. Diabetes, more properly diabetes mellitus, had been identified by the ancient Greeks, Egyptians, and Hindus. In an effort to understand

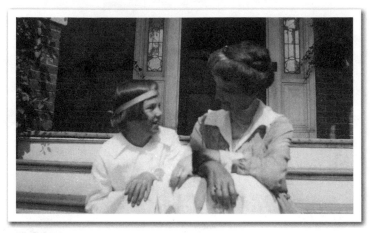

Elizabeth and her mother, Antoinette Hughes, summer 1918.
Courtesy the Thomas Fisher Rare Book Library, University of Toronto.

what was happening, early physicians tasted the urine of their patients and found that it tasted sweet (*mellitus* is the Latin word for "honey-like"). However, identifying the disease and treating it were two very different things. The quest to understand and treat diabetes had been going on for thousands of years to no avail.

But Elizabeth was living at an exciting time in medical research. Significant leaps forward were being made in the field that we know today as endocrinology, the study of the secreting organs and glands. Through these external and internal secretions, the body can self-correct, adjusting, for example, its salt and sugar levels. As knowledge slowly accumulated, even Allen, a pessimist at heart, thought that understanding and curing diabetes was a "feasible experimental problem" that could and would be solved—someday. He hoped that future generations of diabetics would not suffer the way Elizabeth would. In the meantime, his starvation diet was the only means by which she might prolong her life and avoid terrible physical distress.

ALLEN HAD GOOD REASON for thinking that science had the potential to unlock the mysteries of diabetes. Advances in endocrinology meant that by the late 19th century, the field in general and pancreatic research in particular had begun to attract both great minds and money. As early as the 1830s, doctors had made a connection between diabetes and changes in the pancreas, but they were not yet close to understanding how the pancreas functioned. In 1869, a young German medical student named Paul Langerhans identified cells in the pancreas that seemed to be floating in a sea of larger clusters of cells known as acinar cells. Langerhans had no idea what these floating cells did, but because he identified them, they now bear his name: the islets of Langerhans. By the end of the 19th century, researchers were sure that these floating cells produced something that was closely connected to diabetes, if only it could be isolated and identified. Progress toward that goal seemed elusive.

By 1907, the year Elizabeth was born, scientists had begun experimenting with a variety of pancreatic extracts in the hope that when they found the right one, it would open the door to treating, if not curing, diabetes. Biologist Lydia DeWitt, working at the time at the University of Michigan, thought that "probably no organ or tissue of the body has been the subject of more thought or investigation" in recent years than the islets of Langerhans. Scientists experimented on the pancreases of guinea pigs, rabbits, dogs, and cats. German scientist Georg Züelzer gave diabetic patients near death some of his new experimental pancreatic extract; although they felt some short-term improvement, they also experienced vomiting, high fevers, and convulsions before dying. In 1911, a graduate student at the University of Chicago, Ernest Lyman Scott, also saw positive results in his animal experiments, but these also proved to be temporary. The work on pancreatic extracts stalled. Allen, in a landmark 1913 survey of the state of knowledge in diabetic research in general and pancreatic extracts in particular, declared that despite "strong theoretical inducements," all the studies to date indicated that they were at best of "no genuine benefit" and at worst harmful.

Frustrated, some doctors and researchers turned their attention to what might be causing the disease. We know today that it is an autoimmune illness triggered in some as yet undiscovered way by a combination of a genetic predisposition and environmental factors, but Allen and his contemporaries had no idea of the cause. Clinicians tried to make connections to a patient's family history, mental state, or character for clues as to why he or she had developed the illness. Doctors would make notes in patient files such as "healthy life," "never nervous," "regular life: no excesses," "not subject to sore throat or tonsillitis, but has frequent colds with cough," and "practically no alcohol." A few doctors thought that diabetes might be caused by "mental worry" or "extreme nervous shock." Others believed it might be a side effect of the "hardening of the arteries."

However, in the second decade of the 20th century, the search for a pancreatic extract received a boost from an unexpected quarter: improved technology that provided a more efficient test for the presence of sugar in the blood. Up until

1910, urine tests were the most efficient and effective means of determining the levels of unmetabolized glucose in patients or research animals. These were not very accurate and had the additional problem that they reflected sugar levels in the body hours after it might have appeared in the blood. It was possible to measure blood sugar levels but the tests were cumbersome, inaccurate, and required at least 20 cubic centimeters of blood (about four teaspoons) to carry out. Between 1910 and 1920, there were significant advances in technology that allowed fast and accurate blood sugar testing. By 1920, the amount of blood needed for a test had dropped a hundredfold to 0.2 cubic centimeters and the test itself could be done accurately. This improvement enabled researchers to work more efficiently on finding an extract that might treat the disease without ghastly side effects, but the decade yielded no dramatic new results.

Frederick Allen decided to take a very different research approach and experimented with diet as the means to prolong life. The starvation diet he had devised in 1916 was the most successful means by which diabetics could lengthen their lives. He was not the only researcher who experimented with diet. A few years earlier, in July 1912, the *New York Times* reported the work of one group that was sure that *Bacillus bulgaricus,* a harmless bacterium found in milk that is the source of yogurt, might "act directly upon the sugar" in the blood by having a "cleansing effect" on the alimentary canal (the digestive tract). As a result, some doctors encouraged their patients to drink more milk. In 1916, Dr. J. Wallace Beveridge at Cornell Medical School found it "far superior" to using opium, which was given as a balm to patients facing certain death. This research path fell by the wayside when it could not show any sustained benefits. However, Allen's plan did succeed in allowing patients to live longer and more comfortably than any other treatment to date.

In this decade, the Rockefeller Institute was playing an important role in diabetic research. The institute had only recently come to the fore as a locus for the advancement of medical knowledge, but its work had begun with a big splash. It had opened its doors in 1904, endowed by John D. Rockefeller after his grandson died of scarlet fever. Researchers, led by the institute's first director, Simon Flexner, made important early discoveries on effectively treating cerebrospinal meningitis and in identifying the polio virus. These quick triumphs secured the institute's reputation as an important center for medical research. In 1915, Israel Kleiner and his then research partner Samuel Meltzer worked on pancreatic extracts at the Rockefeller Institute until the U.S. entry into World War I distracted them. Frederick Allen was at the institute, too, when he developed his new diet plan.

In Europe, the war brought most European pancreatic research to a halt. Nicolas Paulesco, a well-known Romanian research professor in Bucharest, had begun some experiments on a pancreatic extract but was forced to abandon them in late 1916 when most of Romania was occupied by German troops. At the time that Elizabeth was diagnosed, Paulesco had only just been able to return to work in his laboratory.

Even though none of this activity had resulted in the discovery of a pancreatic extract that could treat diabetes, all the experiments served to close off certain avenues of research and suggest others. This encouraged many to share Allen's view that future years of experiments would ultimately yield results.

IT IS UNLIKELY that Elizabeth's parents knew anything but generalities about these great advances in endocrinology or very much about the physiology of diabetes. However, they could not have been ignorant of what was to come when they heard their daughter's diagnosis. They may well have known people in their social circle who had the disease, as the incidence of "mild" or type 2 diabetes was on the increase. As society became more prosperous, eating heartily and being stout were visible symbols of wealth. "Acute" or type 1 diabetes was also on the increase, but the reason for that is unclear even today. It might have been in part due to the decline in childhood mortality from other diseases. In previous centuries, many children would have died as a result of infectious diseases and illnesses related to poor sanitation. By the end of the 19th century, improved medical knowledge and public health measures that provided clean water and efficiently disposed of sewage had resulted in dramatic improvements in child mortality rates. More children now survived infancy and lived long enough to develop juvenile diabetes. Additionally, making or confirming a diagnosis had become easier. Before the mid-19th century, physicians could do so only by tasting the urine of their patients. If it was sweet, then sugar was spilling into it. Not surprisingly, this was something that many preferred not to try. But in the 1850s a chemical test was developed for detecting sugar, so the rise in cases might simply reflect the fact that doctors were now prepared to test for it.

If the Hugheses had not known anyone in their immediate circle with this illness, the daily newspapers would have informed them about the toll it took in the larger world. It was their habit for Mr. Hughes to read the papers over breakfast and for Mrs. Hughes to read them in the evening. In the news pages and the obituary columns, diabetes was a frequent cause of death for the famous and the infamous all over the world. In 1908, the emperor of China died after a long illness, with his last months complicated by diabetes. At home, diabetes struck down some of Charles Hughes's political allies. In 1902, General Wager Swayne of Ohio, a hero of the Union Army in the Civil War, activist administrator of the Freedman's Bureau, and stalwart of the New York Republican Party, succumbed to the disease at his home. His diabetes entered its final phase in December, when he took a "sinking turn" and died hours later. The disease also claimed some of Hughes's political enemies. In February 1912, New York state senator Thomas F. Grady, an old political nemesis of Hughes, died after being ill for several months with diabetes. Grady was an old-line Democrat, one of the last of the powerful Tammany Hall power brokers from the party's political machine that controlled votes and patronage in New York's ethnic communities. He had personally led the fight against the reform issues Hughes championed when he was governor: gambling, corruption, and insurance fraud. It is unlikely that either of the Hugheses missed Grady's lengthy obituary in the *Times*.

They were probably familiar, then, with diabetes in general. However, they may have been unaware of its different and more dramatic manifestation in young people. Unbeknownst to them, there was one politician whose career the Hugheses would have followed who might have enlightened them. James Havens, a lawyer in Rochester, New York, who was active in Democratic Party politics, had his life profoundly disrupted when diabetes struck his family. Hughes would have become aware of Havens in 1910, when Hughes was the Republican governor of New York. Havens had turned state politics upside down in a special election to fill the seat of a Republican congressman who had died. A deeply entrenched but corrupt Republican machine in Rochester nominated "Boss" George Aldridge for the vacancy. Havens won the Democratic Party's nomination and the election, but he did so by identifying himself with Hughes's integrity and reformist agenda and by drawing many Republicans to his ticket. Hughes followed this drama but was unaware that Havens's life had been transformed in 1915 when his 15-year-old son, Jim, was diagnosed with severe diabetes.

The Hugheses might have been vaguely aware of advances taking place in diabetic research. In the previous decade, there had been an occasional flurry of usually over-optimistic reports in the papers of supposed breakthroughs. There is a strong correlation between mortality trends for a particular disease and press coverage about it. Even if the actual incidence of a disease is low, if death rates from it are trending upward, newspaper reports on it increase. Since mortality rates from diabetes were increasing in the early part of the 20th century, it is not surprising that newspapers were publicizing research advances and treatment innovations.

Many of these reports generated false hope. The 1912 *New York Times* feature article on *Bacillus bulgaricus* had a banner headline that proclaimed "Cure for Dread Diabetes Announced." The fact that this was later proved false went unreported. There was no cure, and death marched on. In 1915, Democratic U.S. senator Benjamin Shively, the second-ranking member of the Senate Foreign Relations Committee, died from diabetes, among many thousands of others whose lives ended without public notice.

ELIZABETH'S PARENTS, THEN, knew what many well-read, educated adults would have known. But what did Elizabeth know about her illness? In keeping with medical practice of the time, Allen did not tell Elizabeth she was going to die. Most doctors at the time, and for many years before and after, felt no obligation to tell their patients, whether children or adults, the truth about their conditions. Today, doctors speak frankly with their patients about their prognosis so that they can make informed choices in the face of new treatment options. They have an interest in patients' rights and a fear of lawsuits. But in the early 20th century, Elizabeth's doctors and nurses felt no obligation or need to tell her what they thought was the truth.

Her parents also never spoke openly with her about it. This was also in keeping with the attitude of many parents at the time. It had not always been that way. One hundred years earlier, it was thought that everyone, even children, needed time and opportunity to prepare themselves spiritually for death, say their good-byes, and pass on helpful thoughts and wishes to friends and relatives. By the time Elizabeth was born, though, many people thought children had to be protected from distressing thoughts of death and dying. Parents kept silent on the subject for their own sake, too. As mortality rates declined for a variety of illnesses in the early part of the 20th century, people became less familiar with the emotional turmoil of grief. Consequently, it became less common to speak openly about death. Elizabeth was never told by her doctor or parents that she was dying.

Without forthright communication from these adults, she had limited sources of information. She could have learned about her destiny from watching what happened to other young diabetics. Modern studies of terminally ill children show that they steadily gain knowledge from other sick children more advanced in their illnesses that they meet in the hospital or online. Through this social contact, they are able to anticipate their own futures and learn the pitfalls of potential treatments.

But this was not a source of information open to Elizabeth. Apart from an initial few weeks in Dr. Allen's clinic, she rarely spent any time there and had no subsequent contact with any diabetic children she met. She never met Jim Havens, who was also under Allen's care. He was now 19 years old and had managed to survive on less than 1,000 calories a day since his diagnosis. He tried to go to college for a while but grew too weak, and became more and more confined to his family home in Rochester. Jim was wasting away and, like many other young diabetics, he was doing so quietly and in private.

Another possible resource for her to learn about diabetes was the newspapers. Like her parents, Elizabeth read them regularly. However, in the period after 1919, news reports on diabetic research were few and far between, and she was too young to take an interest in the obituary pages, which would have been more revealing.

Elizabeth could have asked her nurse, Blanche Burgess, about diabetes. Burgess, who the Hugheses had hired to care for their daughter and monitor her food intake, specialized in diabetes care and had been trained by Elliott Joslin. She and Elizabeth spent many hours alone together. They had lots of opportunity for frank discussions, but she, too, never told Elizabeth she was dying. Burgess wanted to encourage Elizabeth's compliance with the diet and was continuously upbeat about it. She also shared Joslin's view, expressed in his *Diabetic Manual,* that diabetes was not as bad as some other "chronic diseases," meaning that it was not contagious, messy, or "unsightly" like some skin diseases. Her nurse was able to teach Elizabeth a lot about the way her body worked but never divulged her fate.

There was one source to which she could have turned. If Elizabeth had looked up *diabetes* in an encyclopedia at her local library, she would have quickly discovered the truth. She was a regular library user and the 1910 edition of the *Encyclopedia Britannica,* recently transformed from a scholarly book into a popular general reference work, was widely available. It presented the best scientific knowledge of the day about the causes of diabetes and would have been alarming reading. It explained that the illness

... advances comparatively slowly except in the case of young persons, in whom progress is apt to be rapid. The complications are many and serious. It may cause impaired vision by weakening the muscles of accommodation, or by lessening the sensitiveness of the retina to light. Also cataract is very common. Skin affections of all kinds may occur and prove very intractable. Boils, carbuncles, cellulites and gangrene are all apt to occur as life advances. . . . Digestive troubles of all kinds, kidney disease and heart failure due to fatty heart are all of common occurrence. . . . Diabetes is a very fatal form of disease, recovery being extremely rare. Over 50% die of coma, another 25% of phthisis or pneumonia, and the remainder of Bright's disease, cerebral haemorrhage, gangrene, &c. . . . The unfavorable cases are those in which there is a family history of the disease and in which the patient is young.

If Elizabeth ever took a peek at this source, she never let on. However, she might have learned from the encyclopedia that people could die from diabetes but not necessarily have assumed that death from the disease would be her own destiny. Chris Feudtner, a modern medical specialist in palliative care, has suggested that even terminally ill teenagers today, with access to as much information as they might want from clinicians and the Internet, can know that many people die from their illnesses yet not consider that a real possibility for themselves. Elizabeth, then, may well have learned that some people die from diabetes without assuming that this would be her own imminent fate. For this reason and with few other potential sources of information, the efforts of her parents and medical caregivers to protect her from realizing her fate paid off. Elizabeth never knew she was dying.

IF ANYONE COULD HELP Elizabeth prolong her life by a few months, Frederick Allen could. The Hugheses may have read about Allen and his diet plan in 1916 when it was the subject of a lengthy article in the *Times* Sunday magazine. Other diabetologists celebrated the new development. Joslin, in the paper and in his own book on diabetes, enthused that now "acutely fatal diabetes is disappearing." If the Hugheses remembered this news item, they may well have taken Elizabeth to see Allen with some degree of hope. What had not been later reported in the papers was that time quickly proved this optimistic outlook wrong. But the diet did have two very positive side effects. One was that patients, even as they were wasting away and nearing death, experienced a greater sense of physical "comfort and well-being" as they were temporarily freed from many of the symptoms of keto-acidosis. Additionally, as Joslin had noted in the *Times*, the regime liberated patients from "sham treatments" and allowed them a sense of control over their destinies. While several other physicians thought the diet might be too risky and others claimed to have thought of it first, informed physicians conceded that patients were better off being actively engaged with their treatment rather than languishing in "coddled resignation."

When confronted with a diagnosis of diabetes mellitus, then, a patient, or his or her family, faced a terrible decision: either to eat food to try to satisfy the intense feelings of hunger knowing that death would follow in a few months or to eat at a virtual starvation level, waste away, battle debilitating illnesses that preyed on the undernourished, and die sometime later. Elizabeth was never presented with a choice. Her parents made the decision and she was simply told that to treat her illness, she had to stay on this diet.

That was easier said than done. Joslin noted that this treatment "tests the character" because it required "honesty, self-control, and courage." Allen felt that for success (as measured by a prolonged life), patients had to submit themselves totally and faithfully to his plan. And certainly he was able to keep patients alive in a state of "inanition" (that is, starvation) longer than anyone might have imagined. If a hospital stay was not desirable or possible, as in Elizabeth's case, he recommended a supervising nurse. His case notes indicated that without supervision or frequent visits, people found it difficult to stay on such a rigid diet. One adult patient began "eating everything at will" after she left the clinic. Another "lacked the necessary will power" and became "careless in regard to diet and ceased weighing food" even though Allen warned her of the consequences. A male patient might have done well but for his "light-mindedness." Close supervision was essential for success.

However, even patients who stayed in hospitals under a doctor's watchful eye often tried to sneak in food. Both Allen and Joslin found that they simply could not prevent desperate, starving patients from getting hold of contraband. One 12-year-old patient of Allen's, languishing in a terrible physical condition, puzzled the clinicians who continued to find sugar in his blood and urine despite the most stringent monitoring of his food intake. The boy finally admitted to eating toothpaste and birdseed from his canary's cage. This regime was not only hard for the patients but for the medical staff, too, who had to witness their suffering daily. One of Allen's nurses,

Margate Kienast, found it terrible to be confronted by the sight of a starving child and observed that "it would have been unendurable had there not been so many others."

Some diabetics, understanding the general principle, tried to make up their own diet. A popular young journalism professor at Columbia University who became diabetic died quickly of a heart attack in November 1917 after fasting and losing 26 pounds in 30 days. He had continued to work hard at his job even after contracting the disease but told his assistants that he thought "the coming Christmas would be his last." He was right. He did not realize that even the small amount of food that Allen's patients were allowed to eat was carefully thought through. There was already an understanding of basic nutrition science and the food allowed was carefully selected. However, even Allen's patients would have fared better if there had been some means of delivering nutritional supplements, which were not yet available in tablet or any other form. This young man's almost complete fast, not surprisingly, had fatal consequences.

Starvation treatment, hard as it was, represented the best hope for survival, but no diabetologists were under the illusion that this would allow a long life. They simply believed it was the best means of prolonging it. Both Allen and Joslin wrote scathingly of other treatment options such as opium (given to relieve anxiety as patients faced certain death), quack medicine, and one New York doctor's "ham and lettuce" diet. However, all people involved in diabetic care, including researchers, roadside vendors, faith healers, and community doctors and nurses, knew they were simply trying to buy time.

ELIZABETH STAYED AT Allen's clinic for a few weeks to begin her new diet. It was a shocking experience. For the first couple of days, she felt raging hunger but was allowed no food at all. Then, slowly, she was permitted small amounts of certain foods in a careful mix of protein, fat, and carbohydrate, until traces of sugar spilled into her urine. That moment, Elizabeth learned, marked her level of tolerance. Thus, the next day she would have to eat less than that amount. At home in the weeks that followed, she quickly discovered that her tolerance levels varied according to whether she had a cold or was under stress, so she had to learn about her body's responses to certain situations and stimuli. But even once she got into the routine of the diet, there were few periods when, even adjusting for her "fast" days, she averaged more than 850 calories a day. She had to test her urine a couple of times a day and if there was any trace of sugar, she had to cut back her food intake.

This amount of food is well below what is needed for a healthy life. Today, nutrition experts recommend an approximately 2,000-caloric-per-day diet for an 11-year-old girl, about two and a half times what Elizabeth was permitted. Before she became sick, she was a very active child, enjoying tennis and cycling, and she had eaten well to sustain those activities and thrive. If she had been allowed to have the new breakfast cereal, Toasted Corn Flakes, introduced by Will Kellogg to Americans in 1906, and eaten it with milk, she would have consumed about 400 calories. If she had eaten two scrambled eggs on a piece of buttered toast, that also would have been about 400 calories. Such luxuries were now in the past. Oatmeal, an occasional lamb cutlet or egg, and thrice-cooked green vegetables such as spinach and cabbage were now her daily staples.

At Allen's clinic, Elizabeth lived under his iron discipline. But when she went home, she had to rely on her own willpower and self-control. Of course, her mother and nurse watched her like hawks, and that helped keep her on the straight and narrow. The thought of having to report back to Dr. Allen probably also helped her stick to her diet, as she found him intimidating. His manner was reserved, and Elizabeth thought he was like a bulldog in appearance and determination. Yet she trusted him and had faith that the diet would help her feel better. Elizabeth also met Elliott Joslin, and he, too, encouraged her to follow the diet faithfully. In contrast to Allen, he had a warm and optimistic manner, and Elizabeth described him in a letter as just "the sweetest man." Whether intimidated by the stern Allen, wooed by the charming Joslin, or policed by her mother and Blanche Burgess, Elizabeth went home in spring 1919 determined to keep strictly to her diet.

AS SHE DID SO, four Canadian men who would soon meet in Toronto and engage in pancreatic research were busy doing other things. Indeed, they did not yet know one another. One of them, John J. R. Macleod, was already an important figure in the world of diabetic research. Another, James Bertram (Bert) Collip, was a chemist just beginning to do research in the internal secretions of the body. The other two, Frederick Banting and Charles Best, were a long way from even thinking about anything connected to diabetic research.

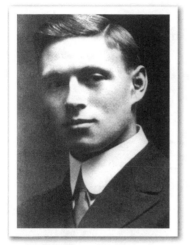

Bert Collip, 1920

Charles Best, 1918

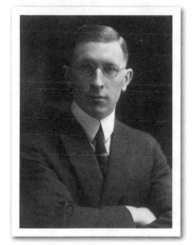

Frederick Banting, 1922

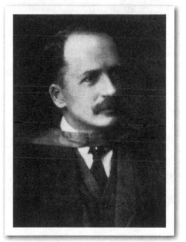

John Macleod, 1923

Courtesy the Thomas Fisher Rare Book Library, University of Toronto.

Bert Collip was the farthest away from Toronto physically. Even though he was a native son of Ontario, in 1919 he was living in Edmonton, where he had moved four years earlier to take up a teaching position at the University of Alberta. The year 1915 had been a hectic one for him, as he not only moved and married his college sweetheart, Ray Ralph, but was also finishing up his doctoral research at the University of Toronto, which focused on blood chemistry. In addition, he was preparing an important publication on the internal secretions of the body. Collip was young to be a university professor. He had entered the university as a shy 15-year-old and was only 22 when he was offered the job in Alberta. By the time of Elizabeth's diagnosis, he was a rising star in the field and enjoying life with Ray and their new baby.

The middle-aged John Macleod was already a prominent figure in academic circles and especially at the University of Toronto. Scottish born and educated, Macleod and his wife, Mary McWalter, were enticed to North America by a job offer he had received from Western Reserve University in Cleveland, Ohio, where he became a specialist in the way the body metabolized carbohydrate. He was hired by the University of Toronto to serve as chair of the physiology department in 1918. The university had by then joined with Toronto General Hospital and become a dynamic place for medical research and teaching, and Macleod was intrigued by the opportunities that offered. He was a prolific scholar, an experienced lecturer, and an able public speaker, and he moved confidently in his new position.

Charles Best, the youngest of the four, was still a teenager, and diabetic research was far from his mind. He was a 19-year-old soldier in a Canadian regiment of horse artillery. He served in the Canadian forces even though he had grown up in the United States, in Pembroke, Maine. His family hailed from Nova

Scotia and could trace their roots back there for generations. Even in Pembroke, the nearest town of any size was in the Canadian province of New Brunswick, so Charley grew up feeling Canadian. A carefree, athletic youth, he began his studies at the University of Toronto in 1916 but withdrew when he was a sophomore to enlist. He was shipped to the Western Front in France but got to Europe just as the war ended. In the spring of 1919, young Best turned 20 and was on his way home. He did have some interest in and knowledge about diabetes, having had an aunt who recently died of it and who, years before, had been a nurse in Elliott Joslin's Boston clinic. However, that connection had not yet translated into any inkling of professional interest.

In 1919, 27-year-old Frederick Banting, another son of Ontario, was also still in khaki and not yet interested in the search for pancreatic extracts. He had enlisted in the Canadian Army in 1917, as soon as he could after earning his medical degree. What Banting called his "very deficient medical training" had been abridged so that all men in his class who were fit could enlist. He got engaged to his girlfriend, Edith Roach, before leaving for Europe, where he served with distinction as a captain in the Medical Corps. In France, he was wounded and received a Military Cross, a high British military honor for courage under fire, at the battle of Cambrai. By the spring of 1919, he was back in Ontario, working in an army hospital, awaiting his military discharge. As he considered his working options, it was the field of orthopedic surgery to which he was drawn, due to both the influence of a good friend and his wartime experience. However, that spring he was much more concerned with two pressing questions: where did he want to make his living, and how long would it take him to make enough money so he could marry Edith? The battle to find pancreatic extracts was being waged by others.

AND SO ELIZABETH began her starvation therapy. Given the challenge she was facing, simply wanting to stick to the diet was not going to be enough. She had to resist the gnawing hunger she felt not only the day she walked out of Allen's clinic but also every waking moment of every subsequent day. She could have withdrawn from the world and lived with her hunger and meager diet as a recluse, but she wanted to enjoy the company of her family and friends. That would mean being with them when they were eating, or at least being in places where food could be acquired somehow. It would mean living a Spartan existence but continuously putting herself in temptation's way. What could comfort her and help her steel herself as she lived like that? What could Elizabeth lean on for strength and solace? She would have to draw on as many different sources as she could. And she was sure she could begin with her loving and supportive family. But she did not know that it would soon be under new pressures that would strain it to the breaking point.

CHAPTER 2

A Good, Obedient Daughter

WHEN ELIZABETH RETURNED home from Frederick Allen's clinic at the end of April 1919, she tried to settle into a routine. She still felt she had enough strength to attend her school in Manhattan, Brearley, then located on Park Avenue and 61st Street. Like many 11-year-olds, she enjoyed the company of her friends, and even though she no longer had the energy to play sports or games, she was a social child and loved to learn, so she drew on her limited store of energy to go to class.

Her efforts to continue at school did not last long. She was vulnerable to infection and often felt very weak. Being called out of class to eat a small portion of food was embarrassing, and sitting with a meager piece of chicken while her friends ate hearty lunches was awkward. She was glad when summer came and she could stay home with her mother and nurse. She did not go back in the fall.

Slowly, Elizabeth learned to live on the Allen plan, getting to know her body's responses to her diet, struggling to cope with the daily hunger that gnawed at her, and trying to be faithful to the regime. She came from a family that put great store on diligence and determination, and she had great willpower. But at exactly the time when she hoped to draw on her family for support, it faced catastrophe and tumult from other sources. Almost as soon as she returned home, her struggle became, in many ways, a solitary one.

BEFORE SHE BECAME SICK, Elizabeth had been fortunate. She had grown up in that happiest of circumstances: a secure, loving, and playful home. She was very attached to her mother, who encouraged her love of books and nature. She adored her father, too, and was proud of his work even though it entailed his frequent absence. She had three siblings, but as she was the youngest by nine years, she had grown up largely without them. The eldest, her brother, Charles, was already a junior at Brown University in Providence, Rhode Island, when she was born. The next, her older sister Helen, had left to go to Vassar, the New York women's college, before Elizabeth was four. Only her sister Catherine had lived with her for any time at home, and even she had gone off to Wellesley College in Massachusetts in 1916 as Elizabeth turned nine.

Elizabeth grew up a happy child, secure in her parents' love. At first glance, neither Charles nor Antoinette Hughes was well equipped to provide such a happy home. Neither had enjoyed a carefree childhood. Charles Evans Hughes had been born in 1862 in Glens Falls, New York, to strict Baptists. His father,

David, was a minister, and both his father and his mother, Mary, hoped that their only son would dedicate his life to the church. His parents saw the threat of sinfulness everywhere and encouraged Charles always to be aware of the state of his soul. After the family moved to New York when he was 11, the young boy diligently studied the classics. In one childhood essay he wrote for his teacher, he explained his belief that "light reading" should be avoided. It would not "educate our moral sense, but will blind, pervert, and weaken it," and so instead he read the books in his father's library on theology and history.

Antoinette Carter Hughes, born in Milwaukee in 1864, did not grow up with much lightheartedness either. Her father, Walter Carter, was a successful attorney and could offer his children a life of material comfort and financial security. But his youngest child, Antoinette, knew little stability. As a baby, she had been christened at her mother's funeral. Because she was an infant in need of nursing, she was separated from her three older siblings and sent to live with a nurse, returning home when her father remarried. Her father's second wife also died after a brief sojourn in the family. Antoinette was dispatched to live with an aunt for several years and then, at age ten, was sent to boarding school for several years more before returning to live with her aunt again. In her mid-teens she returned to her father's home, now in New York City, and another stepmother.

But Antoinette and Charles Hughes also brought more positive experiences to their child rearing. Antoinette's life had been without stability but not without love. She was very attached to her aunt and nurse, and had a warm and respectful if not close relationship to her father and last stepmother. She found solace in books and became a voracious reader, enthusiastically embracing a world of ideas and imagination. Books, albeit not light fiction, filled Charles's life from an early age, too. As an old man, he reflected on the books he had read as a child. He was, he recalled, an "omnivorous" reader and had read "practically all" of Shakespeare's plays by age eight, which he loved "for the stories." Despite this intensive and serious reading, he was always eager for fun and loved going out to play with his friends. His parents may have always suspected the lurking presence of sin in his life, and disciplined him accordingly, but they provided him with love and security. As he grew up, though, he felt suffocated by their vigilance. He remained deeply religious but felt the need to find his own path. He later remembered that as a teenager, his "spirit had begun to flutter in its cage" and he needed to get away and make his own choices.

Both by their own testimony and that of their children and friends, the Hugheses' marriage was one of profound love. Their personal journeys from childhood difficulties had taken them along similar paths. Charles had escaped home by going off to college, first Madison (now Colgate University) in central New York, then Brown, and finally Columbia Law School. He later joined the prestigious New York law firm headed by Walter Carter. He soon became Carter's junior partner and shortly thereafter was smitten by Carter's daughter, Antoinette. Antoinette had just graduated from Wellesley College, where she had fallen in love with art and literature. Now, she fell in love with Charles Hughes.

The couple built a loving home for their children, but Elizabeth and her siblings knew that they were not the center of their parents' world. That place was occupied by Mr. Hughes. He was ambitious, and Antoinette was convinced that her husband was destined for greatness. She realized that he labored under great pressure and organized her household for his comfort and convenience. Their home was to be his refuge. The children were never permitted to disturb their father in his study and they always had to respect his need for quiet.

Both Mr. and Mrs. Hughes subverted their own inclinations in order to advance his career and to serve the public. Another childhood essay of Charles Hughes's spoke to this commitment to the larger world. He had written that real happiness was possible only "by following duty's beckoning finger." Hughes kept this essay among his papers all his life. The couple lived their lives with their commitment to his success and the public welfare completely intertwined. The round of entertaining they sustained, appropriate for their positions both in Albany and in Washington, D.C., they did as a duty. Both would have preferred to stay home together. Antoinette Hughes was naturally shy, although she could exert herself when the occasion required it. Charles Hughes would have preferred to spend his days in solitary pursuits, reading or hiking alone in the mountains, but he, too, put his inclinations aside. His duty lay with his involvement in public affairs. Hers lay in supporting him in that mission.

Hughes's career epitomized this ethic. He was a successful New York lawyer, active in Republican politics, well known for his detailed grasp of complex issues and for his integrity. But he frequently worked so hard that he came close to physical collapse. He was catapulted to fame in 1905 when he was chosen by the New York state legislature to head an investigation into corruption in the gas industry and then later the same year, into insurance fraud. In finding someone to lead these investigations, one state senator, Frederick Stevens, told reporters from the *New York Journal* that the legislature had done a "Diogenes search," referring to the ancient Greek philosopher who searched city streets with a lantern looking in vain for an honest man. Stevens observed simply, "we found an honest man." Ethical conduct and hard work were the cornerstones of Hughes's reputation and success.

With these investigations behind him, high political office beckoned, but Antoinette had to overcome what even the press noticed was a "natural distaste for the spotlight" to play an active role in her husband's campaigns. When he ran for governor in 1906, she rarely accompanied him but did attend lunches or speeches by Republican women, who did not yet have the vote but were making their voices heard. In this, she was no different from other political wives of the time, such as Edith Roosevelt, President Theodore Roosevelt's wife, and William Howard Taft's wife, Helen.

Hughes easily won the governor's race that year and the family moved to the executive mansion in Albany. There the Hughes family lived for the next four years during Mr. Hughes's consecutive two-year terms in office. Investigative journalist Ida Tarbell wondered in the *American Magazine* in 1908 whether Hughes might not have a future in the nation's highest political office. She sang his praises as someone with a "devotion to work," a "passion for democracy," and a commitment to public service. But as governor, Hughes was experiencing enough of the rough and tumble of political life to last him for a while, and he declined to consider a run for the presidency.

Charles Hughes had the public reputation for being an emotional "icicle," but his home was not all dour devotion to duty. It could be playful, too, especially after 1907, when Elizabeth made her own newsworthy debut by becoming the first child ever born in the governor's mansion. Hughes delighted in larking around with his younger children and their menagerie of cats, a dog, a canary, and a pet duck. Even those outside of the family circle discovered that in private he was not the cool, detached person he was in public. An aide to President Taft who had several opportunities to meet with Hughes observed that, when he relaxed, Hughes "was genial, warm, . . . always gracious," and a "witty and humorous man" who loved to tell funny stories.

As in many families, humorous incidents entered family lore. One happened when Taft had visited Governor Hughes in Albany. Elizabeth, almost three years old, had been coached about how to speak to the president of the United States. Like most very young children, she forgot whatever she had been instructed as soon as he arrived. Taft, who weighed more than 300 pounds, took her onto his knee and Elizabeth was alarmed and jumped down, exclaiming, "Oh what a big man!" Fortunately, everyone, including Taft, burst out laughing.

But the years the Hugheses lived in Albany were not smooth sailing. Their social position could not protect them from being buffeted by the scourge of diseases that affected families of all social classes in the early years of the 20th century. Deadly epidemics still regularly swept through communities. As late as 1900, 100 infants out of every 1,000 live births in the United States would die before their first birthday. Deaths of children under five represented more than 30 percent of all deaths. Parents with three children had a 50 percent chance of having one of their children die before age 15. Of course, much of this childhood mortality was not evenly spread through society. Some of it was caused by diseases such as tuberculosis, pneumonia, or diarrhea that preyed especially on children living in poverty, in overcrowded or unsanitary conditions. But other illnesses, such as polio, whooping cough, meningitis, diphtheria, and measles—the panoply of illnesses against which children today are inoculated—did not discriminate among the social classes. The lives of rich and poor children alike could be precarious.

The Hugheses, like many other parents, knew the dangers presented by the two greatest killers of the early 20th century in the United States: tuberculosis and pneumonia. Together they were the cause of death of about 25 percent of those who died in 1900. TB destroys the lung tissue. The visible symptoms are persistent coughing, difficulty breathing, rapid weight loss, and exhaustion. Pneumonia also targets the lungs. It is an infection variously caused by a virus, bacteria, or a fungus that leads to an inflammation of the lungs. Neither of these illnesses could be cured until new drugs became available in the 1940s, and so doctors in the first half of the 20th century were largely unable to do anything to help their patients.

While parents needed to be alert to the symptoms of tuberculosis and pneumonia, epidemics of other childhood diseases swept through communities with deadly regularity. The Hugheses must have watched their children nervously during the local epidemic in New York in 1905–06 of cerebrospinal meningitis (inflammation of the lining of the brain and spinal cord). This strain of meningitis killed three out of four victims.

The Hugheses were fortunate and their children enjoyed good health during this time, but in 1909 their luck seemed to run out. Their eldest, Charlie, now a senior at Brown, contracted this strain of meningitis after the main wave of the epidemic had run its course. When it had taken hold in 1905, nervous New Yorkers had seen the death toll steadily creep upward. There were 104 deaths in one four-day period in early April alone. Public officials could offer no advice to the public, as no one understood how the disease was transmitted. There was also no known treatment. However, by the time the worst of the epidemic was over, a new drug had been developed by Dr. Simon Flexner, director of the Rockefeller Institute. This was a great step forward, but it still left the chance of dying from the disease as one in four.

When news of Charlie's illness arrived, Mrs. Hughes rushed to Providence. She not only wanted to nurse him; she also needed to find a doctor who knew about the new drug. It was difficult to use, as it had to be injected directly into the cerebrospinal fluid multiple times. This was a delicate task and very few practitioners were able to do it. It is a testament to her sophistication and her political clout that she quickly managed to find the only practitioner in New England who knew how to administer the drug. Charlie survived the procedure and made a fast and full recovery.

But Mrs. Hughes was no sooner back in Albany than the family was confronted with another crisis: Mr. Hughes's father suffered a stroke. The Hugheses brought him to Albany, and Mrs. Hughes and the household nursed him until he died a few months later, in December 1909. Thus, within two years of living in the executive mansion, the Hugheses had experienced a birth, a death, and one very close call.

In 1910, Hughes left office and was promptly nominated by Taft to be an associate justice to the United States Supreme Court. Elizabeth was too young to understand the compliment to her father when the Senate confirmed his appointment in five minutes with a unanimous vote. The Hugheses relocated to Washington and now moved in the highest circles of American political life, even after 1912, when the presidency moved from the Republican Taft to the Democrat Woodrow Wilson. Son Charlie's circle was no less rarefied. He had gone on to Harvard Law School, finishing in 1912, and now lived and practiced law in New York. His roommate from Harvard, Francis Sayre, became engaged to Woodrow Wilson's daughter, and Sayre stayed with the Hugheses before the wedding. Afterward, Charlie and Mr. and Mrs. Hughes were invited to an intimate lunch at the White House hosted by the president and first lady, at which Mr. Hughes and Wilson sat side by side.

Despite their many public duties, the Hugheses continued to keep their private lives private. Mrs. Hughes, while friendly and outgoing to her many guests, clammed up the moment she felt someone was asking prying, personal questions. There were some aspects of her public life she enjoyed: she loved fine clothes, dressed beautifully, and shopped accordingly. Many people admired the bright colors she wore, canary yellow or red, which her tall, slender figure could carry off. Both the Hugheses were known as gracious hosts, but there was always a reserve to them and neither made many close friends in the capital.

They also kept their children out of adult concerns. Apart from an occasional appearance by Elizabeth when she was still a swaddled infant, the children were never expected to appear at formal functions. As the older siblings became adults, the rule still applied to Elizabeth. When Charlie married Marjory Stuart, Helen's college roommate from Vassar, in 1914, young children were not invited to the wedding. According to the *New York Times,* the affair was "very small . . . , there being a few more than 100 guests," but it was a society occasion (Marjory being "the first of this year's senior class at Vassar to wed"). Few details escaped the reporter's notice. Helen was the maid of honor and a small army of the bride's college classmates were bridesmaids. Catherine, age 16, also got to dress up, wearing "white lace and a pale pink and white frock." Elizabeth, at seven years of age, was too young to attend. Some matters were not suitable for children.

Too much information was also unnecessary for them. When Mr. Hughes entered national politics, stepping down from the Supreme Court to accept the Republican Party's nomination for the presidency in 1916, Catherine, at age 18, discovered the fact only when she came home from school and had to fight her way through a throng of people to get inside the house. Elizabeth, age eight at the time, was of course also kept in the dark until the news became public.

In this era, families played little role in political campaigns. Elizabeth appeared only briefly at one of her father's engagements. He was giving a speech at an Independence Day celebration in Bridgehampton, Long Island, where the Hugheses had a summer home that year. One of the reasons they were out there in 1916 was because there was an outbreak of polio in New York City. Polio, then called infantile paralysis, attacked the muscles and nervous system. It was only infrequently fatal, but it commonly left its victims permanently weakened and often paralyzed. Not surprisingly, the Hugheses joined many others in fleeing urban centers as the epidemic raged.

Out in the countryside, Elizabeth was able to play freely and her parents could relax before the political campaign began in earnest. On this July fourth, a *Times* reporter saw the eight-year-old Elizabeth at play and described her as one "of the most enthusiastic celebrants of the day." Dressed in red, white, and blue, she looked like "an animated American flag." But that was as close as Elizabeth got to the campaign trail. She was excited about the presidential race. She had amused her parents' dinner guests one night by announcing, "If father is elected and we live in the White House, I can bathe in the fountains!" On election night, early returns indicated that her father had won and Antoinette Hughes woke up her sleepy youngest child, now nine, so she could share the excitement. This was one of the few occasions when Elizabeth's routine was interrupted by her parents' activities. However, this was a false alarm. The family had to go to bed with the presidential race still undecided, and two weeks passed before Hughes conceded defeat to Woodrow Wilson. Apart from this occasion, the Hugheses kept their family life private and orderly. Whatever tumultuous events disturbed her parents' world, Elizabeth was shielded from them.

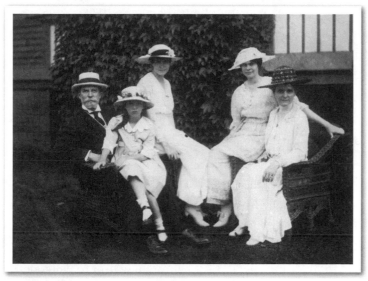

Charles and Antoinette Hughes with Elizabeth, Catherine, and Helen,
summer 1916. Courtesy the Thomas Fisher Rare Book Library, University
of Toronto.

But in the 1916 campaign, Antoinette Hughes broke with tradition. Helen returned home to run the household, freeing up her mother to travel. Mrs. Hughes now accompanied her husband and joined in the relentless handshaking and lunches. In press interviews, Hughes now referred to his wife as his "closest advisor." Yet she declined to express her own opinions on political topics. When a reporter in Chicago pushed her on this, she would only elaborate by hedging. She said, "I have plenty of views on things but I do not like to talk about them. . . . I accept Mr. Hughes' opinion as my own. I am interested in suffrage vitally. So is he, and I agree with him in the matter." Her main duty, she said, lay in making her home "calm and normal" to make her husband's life easier. Still, she could be strong willed. In Butte, Montana, the candidate was scheduled to go on a tour 2,000 feet below ground into a copper mine. When Mrs. Hughes heard she might be excluded on the grounds that it was dangerous, the *Times* reported that she "demanded" she be allowed to go. She was the first wife of a presidential candidate to engage in this kind of campaigning, overcoming her own shyness because she saw it as her duty to her husband and the public good.

By the end of the year, Elizabeth's parents had begun to come to terms with the disappointment of losing the presidency. The family, having lived in Albany and Washington during Elizabeth's life to date, now moved back to New York. Mr. Hughes returned to his New York law firm to work alongside his son and other partners.

This was the world of the Hugheses that Elizabeth now hoped would nurture her as she faced her grave medical crisis. It was a family with a public reputation for hard work, discipline, and unimpeachable integrity. In private, it was loving and playful. It was also one that carefully balanced its private needs with public duty. As Elizabeth came home from Allen's clinic, it was clear that her condition was going to strain these two competing strands in the family's life.

IF, IN THE MONTHS that followed, either Elizabeth or her parents scanned the papers for news of research developments, they were disappointed. If any disease dominated news coverage, it was, unsurprisingly, the deadly influenza epidemic that had reached its height at the end of 1918, killing more than 50 million people worldwide before fading away over the next couple of years. There were no feature stories in the papers that offered any cause for optimism with regard to the "dread diabetes." Perhaps chastened by the false hope generated by *Bacillus bulgaricus* and Allen's treatment plan, newspaper editors did not print any more sensational stories. What little research progress there was stayed in scientific circles.

However, what was there looked promising. After the war, Israel Kleiner, working at the Rockefeller Institute, focused his attention again on diabetes and built on the promising research on dogs he had done with Samuel Meltzer. He first made dogs diabetic by removing their pancreases, then ground up the pancreases, turned them into a solution with salted distilled water, and injected them into the diabetic dogs. By doing so, he was able to see an astonishing 50 percent decline in their blood sugar levels. However, the solution still caused severe side effects. Shortly thereafter, he left the Rockefeller Institute, and he never worked again on this topic.

The following year, 1920, the Romanian Nicolas Paulesco published the early results of his work on the pancreatic extract that he had developed. Unbeknownst to him, he was going down the same lines of inquiry as Kleiner, producing a pancreatic solution in slightly salted water and achieving similar results. These had been accomplished under the most trying circumstances and without modern equipment, so Paulesco was rightly proud of what he had been able to do. Unfortunately, his results, published in Bucharest in French, were not widely read in North America.

The four Canadians had not yet begun their research, and so far only two of them had met. John Macleod at the University of Toronto was settling into his new hometown and job. He had many administrative and teaching responsibilities, though he tried to fit in a game of golf when his busy schedule allowed. He liked working with students, one of whom was Charley Best, now discharged from the army and back in school working on his degree in physiology and biochemistry. Best enjoyed studying under Macleod, whom he described as a "cheery, friendly, highly cultured, very interesting man," although a little shy. In fall 1920, at the beginning of Best's senior year, Macleod offered him a job demonstrating technique and running tutorials for medical students. The young man was flattered and excited to take on these new responsibilities.

Things had been going well for Best. Apart from succeeding academically, he had also been falling in love. He had met Margaret Mahon, a fellow student, before he left for France and, now on his return, the two were seeing a great deal of each other and got engaged in the summer of 1920. That same summer, with work lined up for the fall in Macleod's lab, Best moved out to Georgetown, then a village in the countryside about 30 miles away from the university, where he found work at a golf course at which the best perk was to be able to play a lot. He also joined the local baseball team as the catcher for what became a championship season. Refreshed, he returned for his senior year and planned to do a master's degree under Macleod's direction after his graduation in spring 1921. In the meantime, Best could take things easy. His hard academic work was paying off, his love life was blissful, and his golf game was improving.

Life had not been so kind to Fred Banting. After his military discharge in 1919, he had decided to try his hand at being a general medical practitioner. He headed to southwestern Ontario and set himself up in practice in the town of London, choosing the location because it was home to Western University and near his fiancée, Edith Roach. Things were not going well. Patients were few and far between, and Banting was sinking into debt. He felt restless. To make matters worse, he was not sure whether he should marry Edith, and she appeared to be having second thoughts, too. In need of distraction and money, he took a part-time job demonstrating surgical technique to medical students at Western. He also picked up a few extra hours of work in the research laboratory of one of the university's physiology professors. It was not an auspicious beginning to his medical career.

ELIZABETH, MEANWHILE, settled into her brave new world. The convenient location of her family's Manhattan apartment, on 64th Street just off Madison Avenue, meant that she could still enjoy a few short excursions without exhaustion. With her nurse or her mother, she could easily pass the time in nearby Central Park, the local library on 58th Street, or the Metropolitan Museum of Art about a mile away on Fifth Avenue. Her home was a tranquil place. Her father was immersed in his busy law practice and her siblings had left the nest. Catherine was off at college. Charlie, now with two young sons, lived a short distance away. And Helen was based at home but traveling all over New York with her volunteer work. Still, Elizabeth enjoyed seeing them and her parents as much as everyone's busy schedules allowed.

Her diet went well at first. She was able to eat as much as 1,000 calories on some days. Over one period, she averaged about 750 calories a day. Each week, she ate 1,000 calories for four straight days. These were followed by a day of total fasting, then a "half" day of about 300 calories, and on the seventh day her diet went back up to 1,000 calories. She repeated this for several weeks, with no variation in the kinds of foods she was eating: a solitary egg, sometimes scrambled or made into a sad little omelet, a piece of chicken, and thrice-cooked vegetables, with an occasional glass of milk, which was sometimes made into cocoa if she wanted a treat.

Not surprisingly, her fast days were especially trying but even her half days required careful planning. On those, she perhaps had an egg in the morning, a piece of chicken for lunch, and another egg in the late afternoon or evening. She tried hard to conserve her energy, budgeting her activities carefully. She got in the habit on those days of not breakfasting until midmorning, staying in bed reading until lunch, and saving what energy she had for the afternoon. She then went early to bed after whatever meager supper she might be allowed. Slowly she was getting to know her diet and finding a new rhythm for her days.

BUT, AS SHE DID SO, another potentially deadly illness struck the household. This time it was Helen who was the unlucky victim. In 1918, she was busy doing volunteer work with the Y.W.C.A. and the United War Work Campaign, raising money to support American servicemen. In November, she contracted influenza and was laid low with it at home at the same time as Elizabeth began to experience symptoms of fatigue and weight loss. Helen seemed to recover, but then came down with pneumonia and was ill at home all winter. Both the Hugheses' eldest and youngest daughters were home sick that season. It was only as Elizabeth was diagnosed with diabetes in spring 1919 that Helen felt well enough to return to work. In June, as Elizabeth was getting used to the new diet, Helen was taken ill again when she was up at Lake George, near her father's birthplace of Glens Falls, for a Y.W.C.A. conference. She was now diagnosed with an advanced case of tuberculosis. Two of the four Hughes children had been diagnosed with fatal or potentially fatal illnesses within three months of each other.

By this time, TB was beginning to be understood. In 1882, German biologist Robert Koch had identified the tuberculosis bacterium, and his discovery quickly led to the realization that the disease was transmitted easily by coughing or spitting and thus thrived in overcrowded urban streets and tenement buildings. The only known treatment was isolation and rest. Because it was so infectious, sufferers were encouraged to leave the cities and many people, both in and out of the medical profession, thought that fresh air, a dry climate, and quiet were also desirable. So, people suffering from tuberculosis traveled to a variety of dry or mountainous regions where the air was clean. The need for isolation heightened the social stigma of a disease now associated with poverty. However, in reality, while the disease certainly claimed most victims in dense urban areas, it also afflicted people from every social class, as the Hugheses now knew to their cost.

Seeking the desired rest and fresh, dry air, and with Helen too weak to travel, the Hugheses decided to rent a house in Glens Falls, in the foothills of the Adirondack Mountains.

Mr. Hughes had to stay in the city and could come up only on the weekends, and so Mrs. Hughes arrived with Elizabeth and her nurse in tow to care for their eldest daughter. Two Glens Falls families with whom they were close, the Hoopes and Hydes, found a large house for Mrs. Hughes on Warren Street where they themselves lived. There, they could support Antoinette as much as possible.

Mrs. Hughes spent ten terrible months there watching both daughters waste away: Elizabeth, a diabetic, always hungry but not allowed to eat, and Helen, tubercular, with no appetite for food she desperately needed. Antoinette comforted Helen, who was too exhausted and weak to cough up sputum, the phlegm deep in her tubercular lungs, and Elizabeth did all she could to avoid giving her mother any cause for concern. Perhaps Elizabeth took a turn at reading or chatting to Helen from a safe distance, maintaining hope, as her parents did, that her sister would recover. It was not to be. Helen died on April 18, 1920, at age 28.

The family was grief-stricken. As Helen lay near death, Antoinette Hughes wrote to her husband just after their doctor, the eminent TB specialist Horace Howk, had visited. He told her there was no hope for Helen. Mrs. Hughes confessed to her beloved husband that she had "never struggled with myself more desperately than I have this week, with the result that I have kept up during the day, but the nights have been hideous. I thought after all we went through last summer [Helen's diagnosis] I was prepared for anything but I was not prepared for the definiteness of Dr. Howk's statement." On receipt of this letter from his wife, Charles Hughes broke down and cried.

When a few months later his supporters pressed him to accept his party's nomination again for the presidency, he declined on the grounds that he and his wife were too "heartbroken" to consider it.

Since TB was now associated with poverty, it is possible that the Hugheses and their social circle felt some shame over Helen's death from the disease. The press announcements made no mention of it, noting instead that she died from a "long attack of influenza and pneumonia," clearly not true. A family friend in Washington noted in a letter to an acquaintance that Helen had died as a "direct result of overwork" in the war effort, also not quite the case. However, a few years later, Mr. Hughes was happy to lend his name and his time to organizations connected to tuberculosis awareness and fundraising, indicating that any shame they might have felt had passed.

Diabetes carried no such social stigma. Too little was understood about it, and its victims were equally distributed among social classes and ethnic and racial groups. However, once diagnosed, education and social class mattered a great deal to the meager treatment that was available. Many rural and small-town physicians and their patients would never have heard about the Allen plan. And within the world of diabetes treatment, in which the ability to adhere to a strict diet was central to prolonging life, leading specialists did not approach all patients equally. It was not only that a patient had to be able to pay their high fees; the patient's character mattered, too. The diet required self-control from patients, and Allen, Joslin, and others paid most attention to those who could stick to their diets. These doctors were sympathetic to those who could not do so, but they lavished praise and attention on those who could adhere to the plan and demonstrate its virtues.

Elizabeth's diet records from this period tell of her anguish over the loss of her sister. She had already learned that her tolerance levels fluctuated when she was unwell or under stress, and both affected her now. At the end of March, as Helen lay near death, Elizabeth came down with tonsillitis and was probably barred from Helen's sickroom even if she had the strength to go to it. In the first week of April, Elizabeth began to show traces of sugar in her urine tests most days and her food consumption dropped dramatically to an average of only 400 calories per day. In the second week, continuing to show traces, her food allowance declined to a daily average of about 250 calories, and it moved only slightly above that for the next month. Her body bore silent witness to her grief.

Elizabeth was determined to spare her mother any additional anguish. She never exhibited any of the resentment that some children might feel when their parents give another sibling devoted attention; rather, Elizabeth tried to minimize her mother's anxieties. Indeed she almost sounded like an adult when she wrote a letter to her mother chiding her for being too anxious about her. When she told Antoinette about a problem she had, she wrote, "I hope to goodness now that you won't be silly and go and worry about it." Elizabeth did what she could to make her mother's life easier. Any whining she might have done or cajoling she had needed in those first weeks after she came home from Allen's clinic ended when Mrs. Hughes kept her vigil by Helen's bedside. As everyone grieved, Elizabeth

Elizabeth's diet records, spring 1920. Courtesy the Thomas Fisher Rare Book Library, University of Toronto.

wanted her illness and diet to be one less thing for her parents to worry about. She tried to be, as she wrote some months later, a "good, obedient daughter."

AS ELIZABETH AND her parents struggled with their grief, Fred Banting, feeling sorry for himself and struggling financially, decided to take action to get out of his doldrums. In late 1920, in the course of preparing a lecture that he had to give to students at Western University on carbohydrate metabolism, he picked up a recent article by pathologist Moses Barron that gave him an idea for an experiment. One of the problems diabetes researchers faced as they worked on the pancreas was that the acinar cells performed many functions and no one had been able to isolate those performed by the islets of Langerhans. Autopsies that Barron had performed indicated the islets became isolated naturally after the pancreatic duct was blocked by stones and the acinar cells degenerated. Banting realized he might be able to replicate this surgically and wrote in his notebook: "Ligate [tie off] pancreatic ducts of dogs. Keep dogs alive till acini degenerate leaving Islets. Try to isolate the internal secretion . . ." If only it might be so easy. But to do this experiment he needed a laboratory with adequate funding, animal resources, and skilled staff. None of this was available to him at Western, but one of his mentors there encouraged him to speak to a famous research specialist in carbohydrate metabolism in Toronto.

Banting was excited and wanted to act quickly. He made an appointment to see the illustrious Professor John Macleod on Monday, November 8, 1920. But when he found himself sitting in front of the great man, he was shy and almost tongue-tied. Could Macleod tell that he was broke, in debt, and desperate? Was it possible that change was really in the air? The previous week, the newspapers had reported the landslide election in the United States of President Warren Harding, and it was also a few days before Banting's 29th birthday. It might be an auspicious day.

Macleod was initially unimpressed by the stammering fellow in front of him. He was giving Banting the time of day only because Banting was a university alumnus, and Macleod was not hearing anything that impressed him. The young man was relatively unfamiliar with the scholarship in the field and had no research experience. And he was asking Macleod for significant resources in animals, space, testing facilities, and research assistants, all of which took money. However, after a while, Macleod saw the glimmer of possibility in the proposal. The surgery would be tricky, but Banting had more surgical expertise than most laboratory researchers. It could work and, even if it did not, then at least it would be clear that the acinar cells were more important to the production of the secretion than previously thought, and that by itself would be valuable knowledge. Over the course of several meetings, Macleod became more and more intrigued by the idea.

Despite this generally positive response to his proposal, Banting became less interested in pursuing it. He had felt a buzz of anticipation at the prospect of his first venture into research, but the prospect of a result that simply closed off a research path was not the exciting conclusion for which he was hoping. He considered his career options. Staying put had potential. His work at Western University was going well, and even his practice might ultimately grow. But Banting was definitely inclined to leave town. He and a pal thought seriously about heading off to the Northwest Territory as medical officers with an oil-drilling venture or serving the British Empire in India. His relationship with Edith added to his confusion as she first broke off their engagement and then hinted at reconciliation. Finally, Macleod helped him decide by sending him a letter in late April 1921, confirming that "[u]nless the unforeseen happens, everything will be ready for you here on May 15th." Banting packed his bags and headed for Toronto to find lodgings, get settled, and begin work.

Bert Collip, his wife, Ray, and their now two young daughters were also en route to Toronto in April. Collip had become restless and frustrated at the University of Alberta after being passed over for promotion to department head. To console him, his boss, university president Henry Tory, recommended him for a Rockefeller Foundation fellowship. Collip received the award two weeks after Banting and Macleod had met in November just as he, too, celebrated a birthday, his 28th. Collip planned to spend the first six months of his award with Macleod in Toronto. Tory threw in an extra $1,000 stipend to ease the disappointment of not becoming chair and assured him of a promotion on his return. Bert Collip arrived in Toronto eager to embark on new research.

By late spring 1921, all four of these Canadian scientists now were in the same city at the same institution, optimistic about the varied opportunities that lay before them. Macleod and Best were content with their lots, with both their personal and professional lives going well, and Banting and Collip hoped to kick off the dust of the disappointments that clung to them. It was a time of change for all of them.

LIFE HAD NOT stood still for the Hugheses, either. As the family adjusted to life without Helen, duty called again. Charles Hughes had campaigned on behalf of Warren Harding in the election of 1920 and, after its successful completion, was tapped to be secretary of state. The choice was met with almost universal public approval, and the papers reported that legislators and public officials on both sides of the aisle hailed Hughes as "brilliant" and "one of the ablest Americans in public life." He was formally nominated and confirmed by the Senate on Harding's inauguration day, March 4, 1921, and sworn in the next day. And so the family moved to Washington again, where Antoinette Hughes provided a home for the man she still described in her letters as "the dearest husband in the world." Catherine had now graduated from Wellesley and, when her parents relocated to Washington, she moved in with Charlie and his family in New York, where she could plan a long European tour around her volunteer work. She also wanted to continue her romance with her boyfriend, Chauncey Waddell.

But the move meant that Elizabeth's quiet, regulated New York life came to an end, and her medical crisis deepened. Still, frail as she was, Elizabeth delighted in her father's success and was proud to see her mother by his side. She wrote later to her parents that she always thought she was lucky to have such "marvelous parents." She greatly admired and valued their sense of duty and diligence and their generosity of spirit and humor. She hoped that she shared these qualities. She would need to rely on them to stay on her diet. Ideally, her parents would have been able to offer her their daily support, but Helen's death and her father's appointment changed that. Her family loved her, but they were unable either emotionally or practically to help her at this juncture.

Unlike Helen's illness, during which her mother had cared for and nursed her sick daughter, Elizabeth's care, and indeed her survival, depended on her own efforts. Although surrounded by loving adults, she was, in this essential way, on her own. She had to develop her own resources and interests to give her the strength to carry on. Life had been so busy that she had not had much time to think about what these might be. Now she would have to find out.

CHAPTER 3

A Long Time to Be Away

I F HER BODY WAS any guide, Elizabeth felt more stress over her father's new job than he did. She was delighted and proud of his role as secretary of state and became caught up in unfolding events, but she developed a debilitating ulcerated tooth and had to make drastic cutbacks in her diet to avoid showing traces of sugar in her urine. A few weeks after her father had been sworn in to office, her weight had dropped to 52 pounds. Elizabeth had lost 30 percent of her body weight since her diagnosis.

Still, she enthusiastically stayed abreast of the great issues of the day with which her father was involved. His primary task in his first months in office was negotiating a new peace treaty to end the war between the United States and Germany. The allied powers had signed the Treaty of Versailles in 1919, but the U.S. Senate had not ratified it during Woodrow Wilson's presidency and now the Harding administration also had rejected a key component, the establishment of a League of

Nations. The League, a precursor to the United Nations, was the first international organization dedicated to international cooperation and collective security. Elizabeth was gripped by the ongoing debates.

The Hugheses hoped their youngest daughter would adjust to their new life. The two years since Elizabeth's diagnosis had been tumultuous but now her weight stabilized and she no longer regularly showed traces of sugar in her urine. But when summer came, she was miserable in the heat along with much of Washington. Air conditioning had recently been invented but was limited to a few large industrial facilities and had not yet become common in homes, offices, or businesses. An open window and a fan offered the only possible relief. Usually much of official Washington left town for the season but this year, with Congress in an extra session, government officials and diplomats stayed in town. The Hugheses led an exodus to cooler ground by renting a substantial house, "Greystone," out in Rock Creek Park, at the time on the outskirts of the city. It was on slightly higher ground than downtown and caught whatever breezes the Potomac River could offer. From there, Mr. Hughes could easily be driven to his office and Elizabeth might be comfortable.

However, July proved to be sweltering and even out at Greystone they experienced what Mr. Hughes told his son, Charlie, was "a good taste of Washington weather." Elizabeth wilted, and Mrs. Hughes suggested she take up embroidery to soothe her and pass the time. Elizabeth worked diligently stitching a table cover but, as she later told her mother, by the end of the month she felt that she had done "enough of that sort of thing . . . to last me for years."

The summer had more challenges for Elizabeth than the discomfort of a heat wave. It also had political excitement. Mr. Hughes announced to the nation that he would host a late fall conference on arms limitation, which came to be referred to simply as the Washington Conference, and representatives of the world's great powers were to be invited. In his formal conference invitations reported to the press, Hughes hoped that the meeting would "remove the causes of friction" between the participants and promote peace. Elizabeth knew that she was at the center of pivotal world events. Unfortunately, that kind of excitement was never good for her health.

Her parents realized that she needed somewhere more tranquil, but neither of them was free to leave Washington. They saw no alternative but to send Elizabeth away into the countryside to stay with friends. Although she would not be with strangers, she would be without her family. Elizabeth would have to navigate this new social situation and find her own resources to sustain herself.

ELIZABETH WAS HEADED to a resort area she knew well, the countryside around Glens Falls. She would stay with family friends there, the Hydes and the Hoopeses, who had been so kind during Helen's illness. The Hoopeses had a summer home, "Stillwater," in Bolton Landing, a village on Lake George, about 20 miles north of town, and they would all congregate there. Although the region held recent sad memories of Helen's death, it also had happy associations from many vacations over the years.

In the second week of August, Elizabeth and her nurse, Mrs. Burgess, headed north. Their visit was open-ended and

Elizabeth was to stay as long as she was comfortable doing so. Her departure was noted in the society pages as she set off from the capital but was otherwise without fanfare.

The journey there from Washington was tiring but enjoyable. She and Mrs. Burgess did not stop off in New York to visit Elizabeth's relatives—her brother and his family were out of town on a long summer vacation, and her sister Catherine had already left for a European holiday and was now in Paris—so the two simply changed trains there and continued north. The August weather was surprisingly cool and, once the train left the city, the railroad tracks followed the Hudson River through spectacular scenery. Elizabeth arrived ready to enjoy herself.

Lake George was a wonderful place. The days were warm and the nights were cool, chilly even. The beautiful lake was the center of all kinds of sporting activities. A tiny group of year-round residents was augmented by summer visitors who organized tennis tournaments, regattas, and motorboat races on the lake. Glens Falls, a bustling town of about 16,000 with movie theaters and other urban delights, was within reach should they wish to go there. There were other children staying around the lake with whom Elizabeth could speak even if she did not have the energy to play. There were also sports to watch, if she was not too downhearted by the sight of what she herself could no longer do.

But there were some difficult adjustments to be made. When Elizabeth had visited before she became sick, she had swum, played tennis, gone horseback riding, and played with the others. What would she do now while everyone else was

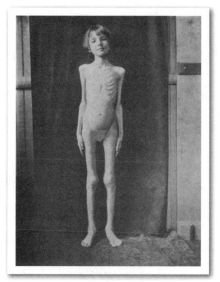

*An unknown, emaciated diabetic girl
aged 14, 1922. Courtesy the Thomas Fisher
Rare Book Library, University of Toronto.*

out enjoying themselves, playing sports and enjoying cookouts on the beach, and without her parents to talk to? As best she could, she joined in. Some sick people embrace their identity as invalids, but Elizabeth never acted or wrote about herself in her letters home to her mother as if she were one. She was determined to live richly at Lake George.

Her friends welcomed her warmly. Often sick people can be shunned or made to feel awkward when they have an altered or unusual appearance, which Elizabeth did by this time. Her hosts had not seen her since she had been in the area when Helen died 15 months earlier. The child they knew then was painfully thin. The girl they now collected from the train was skeletal.

Some sick children withdraw when their families cannot accept either the illness or the physical symptoms of it. However, other children can continue to be social if those around them make them feel valued. Elizabeth's parents clearly did so, and her hosts followed suit. Mary Hoopes and Charlotte Hyde were sisters, daughters of successful Glens Falls industrialist Samuel Pruyn, and their children were about Elizabeth's age. The women easily accommodated Elizabeth's needs and abilities and included her in their social activities whenever possible. In this, they may have taken their cue from the Hugheses or simply acted out of friendship and respect for the family. However, they may well have been responding to Elizabeth herself, who went out of her way, frail as she was, to be an entertaining companion.

The Hoopeses and Hydes were old friends of Elizabeth's parents. The relationship between the Hugheses and the Hydes was especially close. When her parents had events that required them to be in the area, they stayed with the Hydes. As Mr. Hughes noted to Charlie on one occasion when the Hydes had offered to have the Hugheses stay, "they are such good friends of ours that we can be sure they would like us to accept their offer." Elizabeth knew all the adults less well but she was very good friends with Polly Hoopes, two years her senior, and she always had fun around Polly's older brother Sam, who was now 17. Mrs. Hyde was thoughtful and considerate, and Mrs. Hoopes made her large vacation home a place where Elizabeth could find privacy and quiet if she needed it and entertainment if she could enjoy it. Under their watchful eyes and Mrs. Burgess's close attention, Elizabeth embraced the world around her.

SHE WAS ALREADY ADEPT at budgeting her small store of energy to get through each day. Now she had to plan extra carefully around activities or excursions in order to do the things she wanted. When she arrived, she discovered that Polly Hoopes would be arriving two days later. Elizabeth reorganized her diet to have her half day, now 350 calories, before Polly arrived so that she would be eating more and have more strength to enjoy her friend's company when she got there. On another day, her hosts suggested they go to the local county fair at Warrensburg. She was determined not to miss this trip, as it would be her first-ever visit to a fair, but it was also her half day, so she rested completely in the morning before they left to save her strength. It was worth the effort. She told her mother that she "had lots of fun," saw "two thrilling horse races," and "tried my luck at a few things, throwing hoops for things etc. and spent 50 cents—shocking!—but didn't get anything of course." Altogether, she was "much fascinated" by the excursion and had a grand time, so it was worth the planning.

Even on days when she could eat a little more, she organized her activities carefully. In the mornings, she had breakfast in bed. Mrs. Hoopes had bought her a dish warmer ("the kind Helen had") so that her meager breakfast egg would at least stay warm on its journey from the kitchen to her room. Elizabeth often stayed around the house reading or writing letters until it was time for her either to join the others for an excursion or to stroll to the lake with Mrs. Burgess. Her mother worried that these little walks were too much for her, but Elizabeth assured her in a letter that when she rested for a "long time in between it doesn't tire me a particle."

The main challenge of the visit was that she was often part of large gatherings where eating was the central activity, either at dinner in the evening or for picnic lunches. For two years, under her mother's and Mrs. Burgess's watchful eyes, Elizabeth had adhered diligently to the Allen plan and it kept her alive. In that time she had only once strayed, and that was one Thanksgiving when she could not resist taking an extra piece of turkey skin. Mrs. Burgess, the disciplinarian, caught her and gave her a good talking-to. Elizabeth did not forget it. Thereafter she stuck closely to her diet no matter how hard it was. Of course, self-control and discipline were Hughes family values. When the Hugheses accepted the Allen plan for Elizabeth, they were following a treatment choice that fit in with their sense of what they felt she could accomplish. Mrs. Hughes and Mrs. Burgess could control her environment to some degree but could not watch her every moment of the day. Now she was thrust into the world with only Mrs. Burgess to encourage her. Some of the people she would eat with would not be close friends. How would she cope with that challenge?

Surprisingly, Elizabeth seemed to revel in it. She eagerly looked forward to the dinners and picnics, more nurtured by the company than she was tortured by the food that surrounded her. She could have eaten all her meals alone with her nurse and her kind hosts would have demurred. She chose not to. Although she and Mrs. Burgess did picnic alone together on many days, she was occasionally part of larger groups in which her companions consumed large quantities of food. Elizabeth wrote effusively to her mother about these and designated them "red-letter days." She loved the place, was fond of these family friends, and took great delight in the natural world around her. She had many reasons to take genuine pleasure in the excursions.

Elizabeth loved the adventure each outing offered. She described for her mother the picnic organized for her birthday on August 19th as "thrilling." Indeed, she almost ran out of superlatives for it. That day, a Friday, their party drove up to a cabin owned by a friend of Mrs. Hoopes. It was on a hilltop with views of the lake and Vermont's Green Mountains and was appropriately called The Roost. A hired man came with them to carry the picnic materials and build a campfire. Then, Elizabeth gushed, "the most thrilling part of all,—we roasted or broiled our chops on the ends of sticks over it." She did eat the chop, "and honestly a chop never tasted so good," but that was the end of the communal eating. While the others indulged in a spread of sandwiches, salads, and fruit, Elizabeth had only cocoa and baked custard. If this bothered her, her letter gave no indication of it and she described it as a "peachy" day. The group "laughed and talked our heads off" and her friends went out of their way to make it an "absolutely perfect" birthday.

Mrs. Hyde was particularly inspired. She improvised a wonderful birthday cake, emerging from the cabin carrying a decorated round hat box, wrapped in pink paper, and topped with fourteen candles. Elizabeth, frail, took 11 puffs to blow them out and, in keeping with the traditional game, told her mother she would not be marrying for 11 more years. She wrote this with humor, but the timetable was a sad testament to her weak condition. Elizabeth was "completely surprised" at this unexpected treat, but the best was yet to come. When the cover was taken off the box, it was full of presents—two phonograph records from Mrs. Hyde, books from Mrs. Hoopes, and smaller gifts and jokes from the others. Not surprisingly when they returned home in the mid-afternoon, Elizabeth had to rest, but her birthday celebration still was not over. There was a vaudeville show on at the local country club that evening and the whole party went off to enjoy the entertainment. It had been, she wrote, "the most heavenly day I've had in a long time." This was the kind of stress she could live with, and Elizabeth showed no traces of sugar in her urine after this excitement.

Not every picnic was so fun filled, but she reveled in even the more pedestrian meals at which she was surrounded by food and good company. On another day, Elizabeth roasted corn and chops for the others before scrambling her egg on the open fire. Again, her letters indicate no bitterness at this juxtaposition and she seemed genuinely delighted when she exclaimed, "Oh what is more fun than . . . living out-of-doors close to nature." When the group went out again for a "simply corking [great] picnic," a motorboat took them over to an island and they boiled ears of corn in a pail over the fire, then roasted them on sticks. However, the corn was for the others, not Elizabeth. She scrambled her single egg in a specially purchased little frying pan and enjoyed the treat of eating straight from it. She seemed to take pleasure even in the food she was not eating. She told her mother that at the end of this picnic, the group took a walk over the island "after stuffing ourselves enough."

How could she use that figure of speech so carelessly? After two years, she had probably got used to the feelings of hunger. She may also have used her imagination to cope with it.

Children much younger than Elizabeth often resort to imaginative play or imaginary friends to understand a chronic illness or its treatment. Elizabeth was too old for that, but she might have quietly resurrected a comfort toy from earlier years. If she understood her illness as something that was invading her body, as some older children do, she might have seen her diet as an ally or co-conspirator.

Since Elizabeth loved to read nonfiction, she may well have been inspired to stick to her diet by the examples of some of the people she had read about. It is likely that she had read that classic of Western childhood, Alban Butler's *The Lives of the Saints,* or a book like it and learned that throughout history, many people have fasted or denied themselves a favorite food to convey a message. For women particularly, who often had very little control over their lives, renouncing food was empowering. Some nuns and other very religious women felt that fasting helped them identify with Christ's suffering, and others saw it as a courageous act of self-denial.

However, her self-control may also have reflected the female youth culture of the time. Many people were anxious about diet and body shape and had begun dieting. Some did so to fit a fashionable ideal of slenderness. Success made dieters feel proud, as it demonstrated willpower and self-control. In 1918, the first best-selling diet book, Lulu Hunt Peters's *Diet and Health,* arrived in American bookstores, and it had gone through multiple editions by the time Elizabeth enjoyed these picnics. Fashionable women of all ages were beginning to feel the social pressure to conform. Women's magazines and newspapers now contained photographs of slender, stylish women, not the illustrations of an earlier era. Elegant, petite stars of the silent screen such as Mary Pickford and Lillian Gish and fan magazines with real-life tales of glamour cemented the image in popular culture. While there are no records of the other Hughes women dieting, they were all trim. Mr. Hughes admired his wife's youthful figure and she was indeed elegant and slender, despite having had Elizabeth when she was over 40. Catherine and Helen (before she became ill) were also sporty and fit. Even Mr. Hughes considered daily exercise and eating in moderation to be important for good health, and was not stout despite the many formal dinners he attended and more lax standards of physical fitness for men.

It was not only fashion-conscious women who were dieting. Public health officials were anxious for all Americans to improve the quality and reduce the quantity of the food they ate. Doctors, public health policymakers, and social reformers wanted as many people as possible to have what they called "normal" weight. Nutritionists had recently developed new standards for this and used public information campaigns to encourage people to achieve it. In magazines and newspapers they advocated healthful habits of eating and activity. Life insurance companies encouraged their customers to achieve what their actuarial tables predicted were healthy weights. Additionally, to facilitate weight consciousness, penny scales had been introduced around 1900 and quickly became ubiquitous. Doctors' offices and schools often had standard weight and height charts.

Meanwhile, relief agencies were concerned about malnourished children at home and abroad. In 1917, the *New York Times* reported that "one-eighth of all [New York] school children are under-nourished." And news reports from war-torn Europe indicated that more than 2,500,000 children there were going hungry. To combat this, the U.S. Food Administration under its director, Herbert Hoover, had begun a huge relief effort during the war that included encouraging Americans to eat less to allow more food to be exported. Elizabeth may well have seen one of the banners that were hung in public places with slogans such as "Eat Less: Feel Better and Help Win the War."

Elizabeth, then, was not the only person around with anxieties about food and who saw sticking to her diet as a badge of honor. Of course, her situation was both extreme and necessary for her survival. She no longer socialized very much with girls her own age and so was not exposed to peer pressure about diet and size. On the other hand, she did not live in isolation. Sticking to her diet gave her a sense of pride and accomplishment, feelings shared by a number of young girls of the period who had a lot less at stake than she did. And no matter how little food she consumed, Elizabeth never identified her plight with that of children going hungry at home or abroad. Indeed, even sick as she was, she recognized her own circumstances as privileged. She sent letters and money to an orphan in war-torn France that she was connected to through the Girl Scouts. A desire to control her life was the element she shared with her contemporaries. With her well-honed self-discipline, she was able to look forward to picnics for the fun and distraction they offered.

Elizabeth's evenings at the lake mostly passed quietly, with she and Mrs. Burgess joining the others for games of cards or conversation. However, one evening in late August there was a large dinner party, and Elizabeth was so thrilled to attend it that the subject of the food never came up when she told her mother about it. The household was entertaining a special guest, Evangeline Booth, daughter of William Booth, the British Methodist minister who founded the Salvation Army. Evangeline Booth had been active in the Salvation Army from her childhood. When Elizabeth met her, she was commander of the army in the United States and spent her summers at the lake in seclusion to recover from the rigors of her job. Fortunately for Elizabeth, however, Evangeline was a friend of the Hydes and joined the family for the evening.

The party consisted of 14 people, and Elizabeth was awestruck. Part of the enchantment of it was that it was her first grown-up dinner party ("we didn't leave the table until a quarter of nine!"), but it was Booth who made it memorable. Elizabeth told her mother that Booth had "the most winning and strong personality that is positively dangerous to hear her get inspired and talk the way she did last night for you feel as if you wanted to get right up and follow her to the end." Elizabeth referred to this evening as "the night of all nights and I shall never forget it." She had met one of the most dynamic women of her era.

The timing of Booth's visit was perfect, as only that day Elizabeth had been reading Gamaliel Bradford's *Portraits of American Women.* Bradford celebrated the lives of such prominent American historical figures as Abigail Adams and Harriet Beecher Stowe. However, she also included less iconic women such as Mary Lyon, the pioneer of women's education who founded Mount Holyoke College, and Sarah Ripley, a self-taught scholar who was a leading figure in the Unitarian church. These were women who would fit well in the Hughes mold: determined and scholarly, with a strong sense of public service. Dining with Evangeline Booth, Elizabeth had the opportunity to meet such a woman in real life.

The thrill of this evening took her mind off the challenges of collective eating. At the daytime picnics, too, Elizabeth found distractions from the food, but on those occasions it was the beautiful scenery that captivated her. She wrote to her mother in rapturous terms about the sights and sounds that surrounded her. This delight was not surprising as her parents were also nature-lovers, and it gave her a topic about which to write to them. From the moment she arrived at Lake George, Elizabeth made sure her mother knew how much she appreciated the opportunity to see and enjoy its great natural beauty. Much of the terrain was familiar to both of them. When Elizabeth saw a sunset that she felt no words "can adequately describe," she still could not resist penning a few lines of rapture about "the pink glow over the mts [mountains] and reflecting in the water." She then told her mother to "please use your imagination . . . [to picture it] for you know this place so well."

An important part of her love for nature was her pleasure and delight in birds. This was not a new interest but a natural one to develop as she became less mobile, resting for prolonged periods in the garden or beside the lake. Mrs. Hoopes also loved birds and quickly noticed that Elizabeth shared her enthusiasm. On one of the first days of Elizabeth's visit, they had been out on an excursion on which Elizabeth excitedly reported that she "kept seeing *new birds* all the time." Mrs. Hoopes told her about the Audubon Society, an organization dedicated to the protection of, and dissemination of knowledge about, birds. Elizabeth wrote right away to join. She was concerned that her mother might object and so offered to pay for it out of her savings. But, she pleaded, "I certainly hope you won't mind, Mumsey, for it's something that will help me along so much with my bird study, as they send you all sorts of interesting pamphlets about birds and you know how fascinated I am in the work."

She continued to be enchanted by the great variety of birds around her. She saw bald eagles, hawks, wild ducks, great blue herons, and loons. Elizabeth ordered more books from the Audubon Society and knew they would be waiting for her when she returned home. She was ready to start studying "in real earnest and must have the necessary things. I'm getting so thrilled over it for it's a study I can do so easily and there are absolutely no words to express my love for it." She worried that her mother might think her profligate and assured her that she would pay for the additional books "with my allowance."

These were not the only nature books Elizabeth was reading. Mrs. Hoopes had introduced Elizabeth to American nature writer John Burroughs. Her hostess owned a whole set of his works and many other bird and nature books. Elizabeth took some of these out to read by the lake. "I just simply love and am devouring them," she told her mother.

Elizabeth was also pleased to come into contact with less familiar wildlife. She and Mrs. Burgess had the adventure of getting a bat out of their room one night, an event that gave

Elizabeth great pleasure. She was delighted when the bat gave them "a mighty good chase."

For Elizabeth, the beauty of Lake George went beyond the natural world. Her visit there offered her many musical delights, too. Elizabeth had been introduced to classical music, particularly opera, at a young age. On this vacation, she attended recitals by local artists where the standard of performance was very high. One of Elizabeth's most important connections to music was personal and rooted at Lake George.

Her family was great friends with the Homers, who had a summer home at the nearby village of Bolton Landing. Mme. Louise Dilworth Beatty Homer was one of the great contraltos of the age. Homer had, until 1919, been the lead contralto at the New York Metropolitan Opera but had left to perform with the Chicago and other opera companies, although she still performed in New York occasionally. Homer had sung and recorded music with the famous tenor Enrico Caruso, among many other great singers. She had married one of her early voice teachers, Sidney Homer, who was also a successful composer in his own right. The whole family was very musical. The Homers mentored their nephew Samuel Barber, two years older than Elizabeth, who later became a renowned composer. Their oldest daughter, also named Louise, sang too, and twin daughters Katharine and Anne, who were Elizabeth's age, played the piano.

Mme. Homer was a celebrity, and Elizabeth loved to be around her. She was not the only one who felt that way. It was the chance of meeting Homer that had enticed Evangeline Booth out of seclusion and over to dinner. Samuel Barber later remembered his aunt as "one of the most radiant creatures one could imagine." Elizabeth, too, was captivated by her and was quite familiar with her repertoire. But, like Sam Barber, her affection was also based on long-standing association with the family. They were the first people in the neighborhood with whom she had contact when she arrived. The Homer twins came over for a visit before Mrs. Burgess had even unpacked their suitcases. Food was part of the evening, as her guests had come for supper. This could have been difficult but, as Elizabeth explained to Mrs. Hughes, the girls were "so thoughtful about remembering my diet and all" that there was no awkwardness about it.

The three girls had a lot to say to each other. In the spring, the twins had been bridesmaids in their older sister Louise's huge society wedding in New York. With thousands of guests, the police helping to control the throng outside St. Thomas's Church in Manhattan, and the New York elite in attendance (Cornelius Vanderbilt Jr., a former Harvard roommate of the groom, was an usher), the girls had plenty of ground to cover. To add to the romance and excitement of the story, Louise and her new husband had met on vacation the previous summer at Bolton Landing.

Elizabeth had her own news—her move to Washington and observations of society—to share. The girls chatted, played cards all evening, and had a great time. Elizabeth confided to her mother, "I can't tell you how good it seems to talk and play with girls of my own age once more—it's altogether delightful." Not surprisingly, the Homer twins also joined the party at The Roost for Elizabeth's birthday.

Impromptu concerts were part of the Homers' daily life. Within a day or so of Elizabeth's arrival, she had already heard

Mme. Homer sing. A couple of days after that, she went with her hosts to visit them and again Mme. Homer sang. Elizabeth told her mother that she was so excited by this that she "nearly went up in smoke." She pronounced Mme. Homer "just as adorable as ever." On another evening, she went to hear a concert by two local voice teachers, Mr. and Mrs. Reed Miller, and their pupils and sat next to Mme. Homer. Both of them enjoyed the performances. Elizabeth had "a splendid time," but much of the pleasure came from being with Mme. Homer.

Now that she no longer attended school or socialized much with children her own age, Elizabeth had little access to contemporary music. Opera was her and her parents' great love. The birthday phonograph records Mrs. Hyde gave her were opera, parts one and two of the overture to Richard Wagner's *Rienzi,* and she was thrilled to get them. Elizabeth would not yet have heard a radio. That technology was still in its infancy, and in 1921, broadcasting companies were only slowly forming. Wax cylinder phonograph recordings like the ones she had received were generally available, but copies of sheet music still outsold them by a wide margin. So her exposure to popular music was minimal.

Yet she would have had some knowledge of it. Her sister Catherine was one source. An occasional vaudeville show, such as the one she went to on her birthday, was another. Also, the sheet music for the most popular parlor songs, simple tunes easily performed at home, sold millions of copies and became ubiquitous. Songs such as "Bill Bailey, Won't You Please Come Home" and "Happy Days Are Here Again" were hard to avoid. The other young people at the lake also exposed her to dance music. The Hoopeses threw a party in early September for a dozen or so teenagers in their social circle who were leaving to return to school. Elizabeth played phonograph records on a Victrola, an early record player, for the others to dance to. Songs such as "Ain't She Sweet" and "You're the Cream in My Coffee" were popular dance hits, as were a range of songs with new syncopated rhythms. Elizabeth claimed to enjoy the evening and watching the others dance "knowing most of them the way I did." However, apart from these few opportunities and hearing musical accompaniment to silent films on her rare excursions to the movies, Elizabeth had little interest in and minimal exposure to popular music.

The departure of the other children changed the tenor of Elizabeth's visit and left her now entirely in the company of the remaining adults. Fond of them as she was, it was not the same. Mrs. Hoopes had made it clear that Elizabeth could stay as long as she wanted, so she was under no pressure to leave. She decided to enjoy a few more picnics in the early fall warmth.

WHILE ELIZABETH WAS enjoying the pleasures of the Lake George summer, the Toronto researchers were hard at work. The four Canadians had met in May, though Collip and Macleod had quickly set off again, Collip to do some research in marine biology in Cape Cod and New Brunswick and Macleod for a holiday in his native Scotland. Before they left, Macleod offered Banting some technical guidance and made a point of introducing him to Collip. Macleod thought that Collip's expertise in blood chemistry would be useful when Banting came to the point of working on the biochemistry of any extract they might find. Collip was interested in the project and gave Banting his summer contact information in case he could be of use. Macleod had also arranged for Charley Best to work as Banting's research assistant over the summer.

Banting was pleased to get the technical assistance he needed from Macleod and to get going on his project with Best at his side. The two young scientists faced many problems, not the least of which was that they both had to learn much of their experimental technique on the job. Their facilities were good by the standards of the time, but they had to make their lab and surgical facilities ship-shape themselves and continually clean the animal cages in the hot, sticky weather. In the first weeks, Banting ligated the pancreases of some dogs and waited for the cells to degenerate. On other dogs, he removed their pancreases in order to make them diabetic. In this way, he hoped to have both a supply of whatever extract he might be able to create and the diabetic dogs on which to try it out.

Unfortunately, the same heat wave that made Elizabeth uncomfortable at home at Greystone hit Toronto, too. In early July, the working conditions at the lab became difficult. Temperatures in the city stayed in the high 90 degrees Fahrenheit for days and were over 100 degrees in many locations. The high humidity just added to the city's misery. During the day, young Torontonians on school vacation headed for the beaches and cool waters of Lake Ontario. Others sweltered in businesses and homes, and Banting and Best were miserable in their facility. Nighttime offered little relief. City residents, desperate for comfortable places to sleep, headed for the lawns of the city parks. The mayor ordered that the parks, all usually locked at night, were to remain open and instructed the police not to roust anyone they found sleeping there.

Not surprisingly in these conditions, tensions between the two researchers ran high. In one late-night confrontation, Banting vented his frustration, complaining that Best was not meticulous enough. Best seethed for a while but cleaned up the lab, leaving it in pristine condition. Banting had established his authority. While the two settled into a cordial working relationship, it was clearly going to be a long, hot summer.

It was not only the humans at the lab who were struggling to cope with the heat; the dogs were, too. Additionally, some of Banting's attempts at ligation had not worked and had to be redone. As Best later wrote to Macleod using the language of the ex-soldier, they suffered "very heavy casualties." This meant that Banting and Best needed more dogs and had to search the city for them, offering sellers a few dollars for an animal.

They were discreet. Antivivisectionists, people who objected to medical research being performed on live animals, had become active in recent years. In Britain and the United States there were small but vocal animal rights movements. As Banting and Best began work, Dr. Walter Hadwen, a leader of the British antivivisectionist movement, was speaking in New York to support an animal rights bill before the state legislature. The *Toronto Daily Star* carried accounts of his speech, in which he argued that "no one had the right to do evil in the hope that good might come of it." However, these activists had little political influence and the bill was later easily defeated.

There is no evidence that either Banting or Best reflected on this moral dilemma. They needed dogs for their research and went to get them as necessary. They usually identified the dogs they worked on by number, indicating a scientific detachment, although they did give a few of them names. When one animal died, dog 92, a friendly yellow collie with whom they had spent many hours, Banting later remembered weeping over it as one would a pet. However, that reaction may have reflected frustration over the results of the experiment as much as appreciation of the qualities of the animal itself. As Banting and Best went out looking for dogs, the *Star* reported that Canada's first antivivisection society was being formed by a few Torontonians "deeply interested in the subject." Whatever Banting's and Best's feelings on the topic, they were aware that people were sensitive to what they were doing and acted cautiously.

By the end of July, their work had produced some promising results. They had been able to isolate some extract and even though the dogs they gave it to quickly died, their blood sugar levels had dropped first. Both men eagerly wrote separate letters to Macleod on August 9, 1921, to plead their case for more funding to allow the research to continue into the fall. In his letter, Banting addressed him as "Dear Prof. Mcleod." The news in the letter was good enough that Macleod probably overlooked the misspelling of his name.

Both young men were excited about what they had to report. "I have so much to tell you and ask you about," Banting began, "that I scarcely know where to begin. I think you will be pleased when you see how the problem is unrolling from one end and rolling up at the other." The researchers had seen enough of what Best called "fine results" from their new pancreatic extract that they called isletin to want to pursue the line of research. Banting told him they were "eagerly awaiting" Macleod's return to receive his guidance and, of course, assurance of his future financial support.

While they waited for his answer, Banting and Best took a break, swam, and relaxed. Charley and Margaret occasionally went out with Banting and a woman on the staff he was dating (although he was still pining for his ex-fiancée, Edith Roach). Banting could not afford to do very much, though. He was broke. Macleod was paying Charley Best but was providing only equipment and facilities to Banting—no salary. He cadged meals when he could, sometimes from a cousin who lived in town, and sometimes by attending a Sunday-night Bible class where they served supper. However, no one seemed to resent this. He was charming and his friends were generous. Finally, he was even driven to sell some of his medical instruments to raise money. Early in September, before they received Macleod's answer, Banting decided to gamble everything on this project. He sold his house, along with his medical practice in London. There was no going back.

Banting and Best were so excited about the next stage of their work that they decided to begin it without waiting to hear from Macleod. They burned the midnight oil, eating in the lab and snatching sleep when they could, completely engrossed. Finally, at the beginning of September, they received a letter from Macleod. He cautioned them that even though the early results had been encouraging, there could be "no possibility of mistake" and that some might see the results as "not absolutely convincing." However, as to future support, he told Banting that he would "do all in my power to help you" and offered suggestions for refining their experiment.

That guidance was necessary. Banting and Best had not been as meticulous as they could have been. They had not done the same tests or taken the same measurements on each dog, nor could they eliminate other explanations for the results they were seeing. Without that care and attention, they were not only missing data, they were also missing some obvious signposts for paths they might pursue. They had had positive results again from the second round of experiments, but still the dogs died.

Now, everything stalled pending Macleod's return and the authorization to spend significantly more money.

WHILE BANTING AND BEST eagerly awaited the eminent professor's arrival, Elizabeth began to long for home. She did not openly say so. She told her mother she was having a wonderful time and that her hosts' home had become her "second home (don't be jealous)." Even though her parents had just been sailing with the president and Mrs. Harding on the presidential yacht, the USS *Mayflower,* she knew her mother might be missing her. She asked her mother to "promise absolutely to let me know if you get lonely and want me to really come home for some reason or other, for all the heat of Wash[ington] & the tropics put together wouldn't keep me back if I thought that. You'll promise me won't you?" But Mrs. Hughes did not press her to return.

By mid-September, Elizabeth was ready to be home and said so. "Five weeks," she wrote, "is a long time to be away from a home as nice as mine." Even though she thought Mrs. Hoopes was "adorable," it was time for the visit to draw to a close.

The trees were beginning to show their fall colors and the mornings were getting chilly. Elizabeth caught a cold, probably the reason why her daily urine tests now showed traces of sugar. Mrs. Burgess packed their bags, and they said their farewells and traveled home.

Elizabeth's vacation had been good for her. She now weighed about 55 pounds, a small increase over the spring. She had slept well, enjoyed fresh air, and let herself become absorbed in the delights of nature. She had reveled in excursions and found solace in the company of old friends.

Nonetheless, as this frail child waved good-bye to her kind hosts, they must have wondered whether they would ever see her alive again.

Elizabeth had no such thoughts. She could not wait to see her parents and Catherine, who was about to return from Europe, and to catch up on the political news. And she eagerly anticipated coming up to the lake in the future, when she hoped to be able to talk her parents into renting a motorboat and letting her go up joyriding in an airplane. These were delights to look forward to.

CHAPTER 4

Showing Traces All the Time

FREDERICK BANTING STOOD in John Macleod's office unable to believe what he was hearing. Banting and his assistant, Charley Best, had gone to see Macleod as soon as the professor had returned from his holiday in Scotland in late September. The two young men had walked in excited, confident that their summer research had yielded results worthy of his continued investment. But now Macleod was hesitating. The experimental results were indeed promising, but no more so than those of other researchers working in his labs who looked to him for funding. Macleod had to consider everyone's needs.

Banting was outraged. The experimental results had been good—and banking on continued funding, he had sold his house in London, Ontario, and his surgical instruments, gambling everything on being able to follow through with this research. He was so angry that, as Best later remembered, he "began to froth at the mouth."

Macleod quickly relented, although it is not clear whether he was more swayed by Banting's anger or by the project's potential. He found money to pay Best and helped to arrange a university appointment for Banting. Although Banting quickly reverted to cordiality in his dealings with Macleod, the dye was cast for their future stormy relationship.

Banting and Best went back to work. They decided to begin another experiment on diabetic dogs. They wanted to see how the dogs responded to injections of both sugar and the extract but the dogs quickly died, probably from complications from the surgery that had made them diabetic rather than the extract itself. Macleod suggested the two present their accumulated data to an informal university group of students and researchers, the Physiological Journal Club, on Monday, November 14, in the hope that they would get useful feedback.

Banting was not used to public speaking and spent the days before in nervous anticipation. When the Journal Club assembled, Macleod introduced Banting and the research with his usual poise and clarity. Banting's heart sank as he listened to Macleod. The eminent professor was presenting all of the background information that Banting himself had planned to say. Banting was not confident enough to regroup quickly. He stood up and, in a mumbling, shy way, offered some data from the research. Afterward, he obsessed about his own poor performance and, more importantly, Macleod's use of the pronoun "we" when he spoke about the research. The meeting left Banting seething with resentment and marked another step downward in the relationship between the two men.

THE HUGHES FAMILY was having a much better day. If Banting had time to read a newspaper before the meeting, he would have known all about it. Photographs of Charles Evans Hughes and his European counterparts were on the front pages of the *Toronto Star* and major newspapers all over the world reporting the opening ceremonies of the Washington Conference on arms limitation. It was the first such meeting ever. Under a banner headline, the *Star* noted the generally positive reaction of the world's major powers to Hughes's stunning proposal to end the naval arms race among them. It was a key moment in Hughes's career, in the United States' role as an international power, and in world history.

It was also an important weekend in Elizabeth's life. It confirmed for her and her family beyond a shadow of doubt that she was physically unable to stand the stress of Washington life and cemented her parents' decision to send her away for a much longer period of time.

When Elizabeth and Blanche Burgess first returned to the capital from Lake George in mid-September, everyone had been confident that Elizabeth could now cope with its challenges. She was relaxed and looked forward to being home, seeing her parents, and immersing herself again in the comings and goings of Washington's social and political worlds. She even enjoyed the warm city weather. It was a pleasant change from the chilly fall mornings by the lake. There, it had sometimes been as cold as 54 degrees in her room when she woke up. On those days she had a cup of warm cocoa for breakfast, explaining to her mother she would "simply freeze if I didn't." Now, back with her family and rested, she felt ready for the challenges of city life.

That feeling did not last long. The first two weeks after her return, the Hugheses still lived out at Greystone in Rock Creek Park, a little detached from the downtown Washington hustle and bustle, but in early October they moved back to the city. The social season began in earnest, and that, combined with the exciting political times, made it difficult for Elizabeth to stay relaxed. The calmness and good spirits with which she had left Mrs. Hoopes, Mrs. Hyde, and Mme. Homer were a distant memory. She loved being close to the action, but again it began to take a great toll on her.

Her busy parents found it hard to create the environment she needed. They lived in the center of a social whirl. In 1921, Washington was a city of over 400,000, small compared to the capitals of other great industrial powers in the world. The elite Washington diplomatic and political community was even smaller, living in a world unto itself. But the Hugheses were at the pinnacle of this society. An invitation from them was coveted and their every move was watched. The family's permanent home was at 1529 18th Street, just off Dupont Circle at Church Street. Today there are embassies and think tanks in the area's elegant large buildings and town houses, but when the Hugheses moved there it was a residential neighborhood for some of the nation's elite. They were living among friends and colleagues. Mabel Boardman, secretary of the American Red Cross and Republican Party stalwart, was a near neighbor on P and 18th streets. Gilbert Grosvenor, the head of the National Geographic Society, editor of its magazine, and cousin to former president William Howard Taft, was within a stone's throw on 18th Street. Senator Henry Cabot Lodge was two short blocks away to the south and Edwin Denby, the secretary of the navy, a like distance to the north.

Elizabeth knew the area well. While her father had been on the Supreme Court, the family had a house at the corner of 16th and V streets, in the same neighborhood. From there she had been able to walk to her school, Holton-Arms, a private girls' preparatory school, then less than a mile away on S Street. Now, of course, she was not attending school, but she and her nurse could take short walks along familiar streets and her father made the family's car and driver, Charlie Jones, available to them for excursions.

It was just as well that Elizabeth could enjoy the comfortable familiarity of the old neighborhood, because there was little else either restful or private about the daytime hours in the Hughes home. When the family had arrived in March, Mr. Hughes had assumed his public duties and Mrs. Hughes hers. These went far beyond accompanying her husband to formal dinners. The social obligations that fell to Mrs. Hughes were significant. Historically, the contributions of political and diplomatic wives to their husbands' success have been overlooked. It is only in recent years, now that partners are more likely to have competing careers, that governments have offered pay for spousal service. In the 1920s, it was simply assumed that someone in Antoinette Hughes's position would support socially the work of her husband's office.

Mrs. Hughes, like her counterparts, set aside time each week to be "at home" and available to receive guests. People stopping by at any other time would not expect to see the lady of the house but would simply leave a card signaling that the visitor had paid the courtesy of a call. When Antoinette held her first day "at home" after returning to Washington, the household was overwhelmed. More than 1,000 people came, some just to leave their cards, others hoping to meet Mrs. Hughes. Not surprisingly, she ran out of food!

Of course, she had been part of this well-established social machine before and, after this initial tidal wave of guests, she settled into the routine. On Monday afternoons, wives of Supreme Court justices were at home to visitors. On Wednesdays, it was the turn of the cabinet wives. On Fridays, the wives of foreign ambassadors and other diplomats received guests. Of course, on all these days everyone else was doing the visiting or leaving cards.

If Elizabeth had been healthy, she would have been away from the house for much of this activity, occupied with school and sports. Now, when Wednesday afternoons came, she stayed out of the way, joining in only when someone she knew or particularly wanted to meet was coming. Still, she enjoyed hearing the news from her mother afterward.

This social activity by itself would not have left Antoinette much time to sit at home with Elizabeth, and the regular visiting calendar was just a small part of her obligations. She had an extensive correspondence to maintain. She took an interest in and lent her name to organizations whose work she supported, such as the Columbia Hospital for Women and the International Relationships Committee of the General Federation of Women's Clubs. And, of course, all this public and private entertaining meant many an hour spent with dressmakers and milliners. The newspaper society pages described her clothing in detail whenever she made public appearances. She had to look good. As she aged, Mrs. Hughes eschewed some of the dazzling colors she had worn when she was younger. Now, she favored softer colors such as ivory, or rose with sequins and other decoration for evening wear, but she continued to wear bolder colors and styles, stripes, or geometric designs during the day.

In the fall of 1921, the most time-consuming of these many social responsibilities was the planning for the Washington conference, set to convene on Saturday, November 12, the day after the Armistice ceremonies marking the anniversary of the end of the recent World War. Mrs. Hughes was not involved in the logistical details of the conference business, the minutia of etiquette involving the nine invited nations, the four delegates from each, and the advisors that they brought with them. But she was involved in the planning of the conference's principal social event: a grand evening reception that she and her husband would host on Monday, November 14. It was to be held in the Hall of the Americas at the Pan American Union building, now the home of the Organization of American States, on 17th Street N.W., a short distance from the Washington Monument. The guest list numbered more than 2,000 people and the leading lights of Washington's social, political, and diplomatic circles were invited, along with the visiting conference delegations. Not surprisingly, planning it was hard work for the State Department, Antoinette Hughes, and her secretary. Even daughter Catherine, otherwise dividing her time between Washington and New York, was drafted into helping.

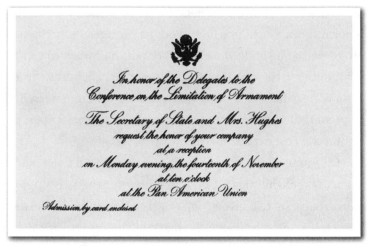

Invitation to the Hugheses' reception to celebrate the opening of the Washington Conference. Courtesy Library of Congress.

Their hard work paid off. It was the grand event of the Washington season. The *Washington Post* reported that Mrs. Hughes, wearing a deep rose satin gown, with "festoons of crystal on the bodice and the skirt" set off with a simple black headband and diamond clasp, stood beside Secretary Hughes. They received their guests personally at the top of a grand staircase, the introductions made by a White House military aide. The hall was packed with men in evening dress or uniforms and women in "elegant gowns and splendid jewels." The building looked its best, too. The exterior was decorated with lights and inside, flowers, silk flags, and more unusual illuminations covered the marble halls. It was, everyone agreed, "a brilliant reception."

The weekend had been a crowning achievement for Secretary Hughes. Two days earlier, the opening ceremony was appropriately grand and his welcoming speech, which contained bold new policy initiatives to limit naval power, created a sensation. Everyone who was anyone in Washington society was present. Mrs. Hughes sat next to Vice President Calvin Coolidge. Alice Roosevelt Longworth, the daughter of former president Theodore Roosevelt and wife of Ohio congressman Nicholas Longworth, was nearby, as were William Howard Taft, recently appointed as chief justice of the Supreme Court, his wife, Helen, and many other dignitaries.

Socially and politically, it was an exhausting long weekend. As the *Post* observed a few days later, many society hostesses, confronted by the "multitude of entertainments" around the conference, found the evening gowns in their possession to be inadequate and were "busily adding to these wardrobes." Many evenings involved multiple events, with the glitterati noticing not only the fashions but also who dined with whom and who was moving up or down the social pecking order.

And the conference was just the beginning of the fall social season. Within three weeks, many of the political and diplomatic set were wilting under the strain. The cabinet members' wives banded together and announced that they were curtailing their visiting. The wives of the more junior ministers, who lived near one another in the Wardman Park area (near the National Zoo, a mile or so away from Dupont Circle), announced they would receive visitors together at one of their homes to streamline the task. The more senior—Mrs. Hughes, together with Mrs. Hoover, Mrs. Denby, and Mrs. Weeks (the wives of the secretaries of Commerce, Navy, and War, respectively)—announced that they would be "at home" only the first Wednesday of each month, sharply curtailing the time they were available to receive guests. But still, the pace of entertaining remained hectic.

Elizabeth knew it was a thrilling period in her father's life and the country's history and loved hearing all the details. Although she was not directly involved in this whirlwind, she was caught up in the excitement of what she called "a wild wonderful historic" time, and her diet suffered as a result. She was, she wrote a few weeks later, "showing traces all the time." She had to reduce her food intake sharply in order to stay below her tolerance levels. While she knew this was happening because of her eager interest in the conference and its social activities, she "wouldn't have missed it for anything."

But something had to give. The Hugheses agonized over how best to care for their daughter, but they were quite sure where their duty lay. They loved their children but they must have felt that at age 60, Mr. Hughes's senior cabinet position was likely to be the most important work he would ever do. For an ambitious couple who celebrated public service as a duty and an honor, they felt that this job, which would allow him to use his talents on the world stage, would be the pinnacle of a life lived in the service of the law, his community, and the nation. The planning and successful commencement of the conference confirmed that sense of purpose.

There is no record of the Hugheses' deliberations over what to do about Elizabeth and it is unlikely she was ever involved in the discussion. Given their commitment to Mr. Hughes's job, their options were few. Mrs. Hughes could have been more public about Elizabeth's illness and offered it as an excuse not to participate in the social world of Washington. People would have been sympathetic. But such a course went against the family's strong inclination for privacy and her own desire to support her husband as much as possible. She could have left town and sequestered herself somewhere with Elizabeth, as she had done when she had nursed Helen and before her husband's new job. But both these options would have left her unable to stand at her husband's side literally and figuratively. Mr. Hughes needed the woman he called his "strong loyal wife" at his side, and she wanted to be there.

Their solution, probably arrived at in the days immediately before the opening of the conference, was to send Elizabeth away again. This time, they decided that she and Mrs. Burgess would travel hundreds of miles away and be gone for six months. Their destination would be the British island colony of Bermuda.

IT WAS A WISE CHOICE. If there was a place that might offer Elizabeth tranquility, it was Bermuda, a place famous for its beauty and slow pace of life. Located on the same latitude as Charleston, South Carolina, the tightly packed group of islands that make up Bermuda is about 770 miles southeast of New York and 590 miles east southeast of Cape Hatteras, North Carolina. Its temperate winter climate averages about 63 degrees and even though the humidity can be high, there is a permanent cool breeze and abundant sunshine.

The country was already a great favorite with wealthy American tourists. According to the *New York Times,* a record 30,000 of them would travel to the island in the winter of

1921, overwhelming the island's permanent population of about 20,000. Given that the closely nestled islands totaled only 21 square miles, it was already densely populated, but one did not need to move too far away from the small capital, Hamilton, to enjoy peace and quiet. Bermuda had banned the automobile, believing its lanes too narrow for motor traffic, adding to its tranquility. While an enthusiastic group of island residents regularly lobbied for that to change, most tourists found horse-and-cart transportation charming and liked the slower pace of life that it dictated.

The Hugheses themselves had never been to Bermuda but people in their social circle had. They also knew about the place from many other sources. Indeed, feature articles and news stories about Bermuda were so common that it would have been hard for them not to have known a good deal about it. For more than a century it had been a British naval supply base, and during the American Civil War it was a place notorious for harboring Confederate blockade runners. In 1888, the inauguration of regular steamship and mail services from New York led to a surge in tourism. Even the British decision at the end of the century to hold prisoners from the South African (Boer) War on the islands did not slow the steady increase in American visitors. By the end of the first decade of the 20th century, more than 9,000 of them annually traveled there.

Over these years, there had been a steady outpouring of newsy articles about the islands' delights. Among them were *New York Times* correspondent William Drysdale's breezy accounts of Bermudian life. William Dean Howells supplied the same in *Harper's Magazine,* and Mark Twain wrote an entertaining story of his Bermudian travels in his book *The Stolen White Elephant and Other Detective Stories.*

As the years passed and the number of tourists increased, the island could still offer tranquility, but it also now had its own winter social season as wealthy visitors jammed the few hotels with dinners, parties, and dances. The social activities of celebrities such as Mrs. John Barrymore, wife of the famous silent-screen actor, made the front pages of the local paper. Other visitors were equally well known but more discreet. Woodrow Wilson, before he became president, played golf there and began his friendship with the flirtatious and lovely Mary Peck. William and Helen Taft had also visited the resort only a few months before Elizabeth set sail.

How much did she know about the place to which she was being dispatched? Elizabeth would certainly have acquired a guidebook. There were plenty to choose from, such as *Bermuda Past and Present, Beautiful Bermuda,* or *Rider's Bermuda,* which came out while she was there. This was a relatively new genre and these books were filled with the kind of information that would be familiar to modern travelers: details about the history and natural history of the place, restaurants and transportation, the resources of Hamilton, the customs of the area, and the most scenic places to visit.

The technology was not yet available to allow these books to reproduce photographs easily or cheaply, so there were few illustrations in them, other than maps, to help Elizabeth imagine the place before she set foot on it. However, she may have seen vacation photos from family friends. These were a new phenomenon. The Eastman Kodak Brownie box camera had

been introduced only in 1900, and George Eastman had to educate people in the ways they might use it. He encouraged them
to take a snapshot, a picture that caught an activity or moment
in time, rather than a formal, posed portrait. The cameras were
roughly three inches by three inches by five inches, small and
portable compared to earlier ones. By the time Elizabeth and
Mrs. Burgess set off on their trip, the Kodak box camera and
its competitors were ubiquitous. Elizabeth loved hers, and she
and her friends took many vacation photographs.

Winslow Homer's paintings of Bermuda would have given
her an idea of the island's delights. Many of those were exhibited in New York during the years she lived there. The family's
apartment on East 64th Street was just a few short blocks away
from Babcocks, a gallery at 47th Street and Fifth Avenue, and
the Anderson Galleries on Park Avenue and 57th Street, where
his work was shown and sold. Homer captured the clear blue
skies, distinctive whitewashed buildings, and small scudding
clouds familiar to island visitors and residents.

If she had not seen these paintings or photographs, then,
like many travelers before her, Elizabeth would have had to
set off with only the descriptions of others to stimulate her
imagination, and there had been plenty of that recently available. Because writers often found it hard to find words to cap-
ture the unique beauties of Bermuda, many of them relied on
Mark Twain. He had consciously struggled to find the right
vocabulary, especially to describe the buildings. The houses
there, including the roofs, were made of the white coral sandstone indigenous to the island. The sandstone was then whitewashed, leaving it sparkling in the sunshine. Twain noted that

he and his traveling companion had to "put in a great deal of solid talk and reflection" toward getting the description right. They concluded that the buildings were "the white of the icing of a cake" and, indeed, "too pure and white for this world."

Elizabeth could have easily found Twain's book, but there had also been a recent article in *Vogue* (a must-read for society households) describing the resort, celebrating its beauty, tranquility, and the "delightful balls and garden parties" of the social season. And she may have spoken to the Tafts. They loved the place and on the couple's return from Bermuda earlier that year, former president Taft had given a talk to the National Geographic Society detailing his impressions of the place and its history. He had quoted Twain and added his own general celebration of the "luxuriance and wealth of color" in the surroundings and "philosophic contentment" of its peoples.

Elizabeth and Mrs. Burgess set off the first week of December 1921 as the mild late fall weather turned to winter chill. Mrs. Burgess packed their bags and Elizabeth made sure her camera was safely stowed. The journey was tiring. The steamship companies that vied with each other for the tourist dollar operated only out of New York, so Elizabeth and Mrs. Burgess first had to get there by train. As they left Washington, the papers alerted travelers to bad weather off Cape Hatteras. An early winter storm was moving northeast. But the steamship companies kept to their schedules in fair weather or foul. The two transferred to their ship, the *Fort Hamilton,* in New York and settled into their cabin for the 45-hour voyage to Hamilton.

It could have been a miserable journey but, as Elizabeth later told her mother, the two were lucky. Their cabin, number 18, was in the more stable middle of the ship, and Mrs. Burgess had an "exceedingly good preventative for seasickness." This was to take Epsom salts (magnesium sulfate, a mild laxative among its many other uses) in the morning the day before they sailed, followed by two doses of calomel (mercurous chloride, a stronger laxative and diuretic) the night before sailing. Mrs. Burgess was sure these two combined would prepare the body for the rough seas they might face. It worked, and they spent an enjoyable voyage looking forward to the delights of Bermuda.

BY EARLY DECEMBER 1921, Charley Best, Banting's young research partner, probably wished that he could find an Atlantic island that offered him a calm retreat. He was an easygoing, affable young man, and it was sometimes difficult for him to juggle the strong personalities around him and the ups and downs of the research journey. He was aware of the tensions arising from the Journal Club meeting and tried to keep his head down.

Despite the difficulties of that day, some positive developments came out of it. One person at the meeting suggested they do a longevity study to see how long a diabetic dog could be kept alive on their extract, advice they decided to follow. Earlier experiments had focused only on the extract's immediate effects; the goal now would be to see whether giving it on a regular schedule would prolong a diabetic animal's life. Another outcome was that word began to spread on the academic grapevine that some interesting developments were taking place. Elliott Joslin heard about the research and wrote to Macleod to ask if there was even "a grain of hopefulness" that he could pass on to any of his desperately sick patients. In his reply, Macleod gave him only that grain: they had found something "that may be of real value," but they were still a long way away from human clinical trials. Word also spread to George Clowes, the research director of the Indianapolis drug company Eli Lilly & Company, who decided to follow the progress of the Toronto research.

At that moment, there was little progress going on for him to follow. As Banting and Best began to design the longevity experiment, they realized how hampered they were by the slow and difficult means by which they were gleaning the extract—by pursuing Banting's original research idea of ligating healthy dogs and waiting for the acinar cells to degenerate. They tried to think of other ways they might acquire it.

They then made two important discoveries in quick succession. Scientists already knew that the islets of Langerhans, the cells in the pancreas that seemed to be the source of the problem for diabetics, were especially plentiful in the pancreases of fetal and newborn animals. Using cattle fetuses from a local slaughterhouse, they confirmed that the islets and the internal secretion they produced were indeed plentiful. But Banting and Best also discovered something else. The pancreas produces other excretions that facilitate digestion but since digestion begins after birth, they realized the internal secretion in the fetus was pure. Now they had a faster means of securing a supply of the extract.

Then, by following a suggestion of Macleod's, they found a means of increasing the supply yet more. They discovered that they could derive the extract by making a solution of a ground whole cattle pancreas with alcohol. There had never been any need for the unusual and creative avenues they had pursued.

Now, with a steady supply of extract, the experimental work moved forward rapidly. They could try out new preparations and delivery techniques to find, for example, how much the extract should be filtered, whether it should be boiled, how concentrated it should be, and whether it could be delivered directly into the stomach or needed to be injected.

In early December, Macleod decided that it was time for Collip to join the group. Collip was a skilled and creative biochemist, and he quickly made improvements to the technique of producing the extract in a solution of alcohol. He also dissected a treated dog and demonstrated that the extract was restoring important metabolic functions in the liver. For those suffering from diabetes, ketones in the liver reach toxic levels as the body responds to a shortage of glucose, leading to organ failure. He saw that the extract eliminated ketones and restored glycogen. Excited about his discovery, Collip headed home to his wife and children for Christmas celebrations. Banting and Best were pleased, too. If they were bothered by the fact that it was Collip and not they who had made this discovery, they kept their disappointment to themselves.

Even though there had not yet been one animal survivor of their longevity studies, Banting was eager to move to human trials. Shortly before Christmas, probably without Macleod or Collip's knowledge, he called an old medical school classmate in Toronto, Joseph Gilchrist, who was wasting away from acute diabetes, prolonging his life on Allen's plan. Banting told him what the group was working on and Gilchrist volunteered to try some of the extract. Banting, perhaps remembering the fate of some of the dogs, was cautious and gave his friend the treatment orally. (Banting did not know yet that when taken by mouth, digestive enzymes would break down the extract, making it useless.) Fortunately for Gilchrist, he suffered no bad effects, but he received no benefits either.

The pace and range of the research was now advancing rapidly. Everyone was in better spirits, and the four met regularly to discuss their work. They planned to take the train down to Yale University in New Haven, Connecticut, immediately after the holidays, where several weeks before they had arranged to present their work at the American Physiological Society conference on December 30. But first, they each went home to feast and rest for a couple of days. The research team had not found anything like Bermudian tranquility, but they had stopped arguing and the work was going well.

ELIZABETH AND MRS. BURGESS settled into "Honeymoon Cottage" in Pembroke Parish, just outside Hamilton. The Hugheses had rented the small house through an agent the week of their glittering reception in the Pan American Union building. As her parents waved her off a couple of weeks later, they may have felt some guilt over their decision to send their daughter away. Mrs. Hughes perhaps particularly did so, but her place was where it had always been, at her adored husband's side. Also, having nursed and watched as Helen approached death, she probably dreaded the tests that again lay ahead of her. As their eldest daughter was dying, Antoinette had written to her husband that all the thoughts that rushed through her mind "nearly drove me mad." Perhaps the memory of that made the decision to send Elizabeth away an easier one.

Elizabeth's letters never hint at any resentment at this, but it is unlikely that she was open about how she felt either in person or in her letters home. Dying children and their families often engage in a mutual pretense about how fine everything is. It is a common coping mechanism that parents and children employ to get through a crisis and avoid speaking about the reality of the situation. It keeps the world orderly and manageable, a strategy that was probably appealing in a disciplined family such as the Hugheses. When the children do not know they are dying but the adults around them do, as in Elizabeth's case, the adults' forced cheerfulness and "business as usual" attitude is an attempt to shield the children from their bleak reality, and the children come to mirror the adults' positive demeanor. A determination to be cheerful and to follow life's usual activities as much as possible was the order of the day, and Elizabeth followed it.

Business as usual in the Hughes household had revolved around her father's needs since before Elizabeth was born. She had been raised to value and admire his work. From Bermuda, she told her mother that she "realize[d] fully the demands on Father" and understood that those demands took precedence. She was also quite used to being away from her parents. Like children in other elite families, she had been cared for by a nanny or other domestic help in her earliest years. As the Hugheses had always had extensive public and social commitments, she had spent many days and evenings in the company of an adult outside the family circle. In the months since her father became secretary of state, she had spent a good deal of time alone with her nurse long before the two were sent away.

Elizabeth also recognized her own need to be away from the excitement of Washington. Much as she had been thrilled by all the conference activities, she had paid a high price for it with days of being allowed to eat only 200 or 300 calories in order to avoid sugar spilling into her urine. She told her mother, "I don't want another excitement like it to upset me again."

So the travelers settled into Honeymoon Cottage and made themselves at home. They found some evergreens to drape across the fireplace to serve as Christmas decorations, made the room cozy, and took a snapshot of it on Christmas morning. Elizabeth sent the photograph to her mother. "[I]t's the 1st 'interior' I've ever taken & I am quite proud of it," she told her. But there could be no special holiday foods. Elizabeth consumed only 800 calories that day. And there was no Mrs. Hyde to think up a creative, festive surprise. Elizabeth and Mrs. Burgess sat down together but to different meals and marked the holiday quietly, a long way from home. Elizabeth must have wondered what the New Year would bring but could not imagine the great trials—and surprising pleasures—that lay ahead of her.

CHAPTER 5

How I Do Love Writing

O NE SUNDAY EVENING in early January 1922, Elizabeth sat down in front of a cozy fire in Honeymoon Cottage to write to her mother. But before she began recounting the day's events, she had to vent.

She had recently visited several of her mother's Washington society friends: Mrs. Sadie Gaff, wife of Thomas Gaff, a wealthy businessman and industrialist, who lived in a grand mansion on 20th and Q streets; Mrs. Huybertie Hamlin and her adult daughter, Anna, the family of Charles Hamlin, a former chairman of the Federal Reserve Board, near neighbors over on New Hampshire Avenue; and on this particular sunny afternoon, one Mrs. Oliver, vacationing near the Bermudian South Shore. Elizabeth enjoyed the get-together well enough—or claimed to—but she had had enough. She decided to protest:

> I didn't come to Bermuda to go to teas and go calling on
> your friends every minute ... and although they're all sweet

& all & I like to visit with them, still can't you imagine my
position somewhat, & can't you see what a bore & nui-
sance it is for I really ought to return their calls, I suppose?
I thought after I'd seen them all once or twice it would be
enough, but heavens they keep on pestering the life out of
me and I don't know what to do, for I simply detest spending all these lovely aft[ernoons] dressing up & calling on old
ladies, pardon me, but they do seem old for a girl of 14 to
keep up with all the time. Please, please pity me....

Of course, Elizabeth was making a tactical error. Had
she pleaded exhaustion, her mother would have relented.
Mrs. Hughes was concerned that her daughter was trying to
do too much on her meager food intake. But instead Elizabeth
argued that it simply interfered with her ability to enjoy herself.
She went on, digging herself into a deeper hole:

we always have to rent a carriage (which is no small matter, we find down here) & we've been spending quite a bit
doing that lately ... We endeavor to keep our carriage bills
down, only using them for special trips & long picnics & to
sight-see etc. But it seems absurd to spend so much for just
calling. Oh the whole thing makes me mad & I just simply
had to tell you from the "bottom of my heart" what I really
thought & how I could manage to abolish it. Do write and
tell me soon, won't you, as they're your friends?

Mrs. Hughes was unsympathetic—and not just because
these women were her age or younger. She did not tolerate

whining, and especially not about a social obligation as important as visiting.

However, her response was probably more complicated than that. On the one hand, it was comforting to have her daughter behave as a normal teenager. But parents of dying children are often torn over whether to require the usual responsibilities from them. They are tempted to be overindulgent but they also have to live with the child, sometimes for a prolonged period, so they keep to their usual expectations but feel guilty about it. The Hugheses had always guided Elizabeth with a loving but firm hand. Now, she was a sick child but not a spoiled one. As long as she was able, her parents expected her to be socially engaged. Mrs. Hughes was unmoved by her daughter's complaint. Elizabeth never raised the subject again and continued visiting and receiving guests in turn.

One afternoon, Elizabeth and Mrs. Burgess went to see Mrs. Hamlin and her daughter Anna, who had just turned 21. "Little Elizabeth Hughes at tea," Anna noted in her diary. She thought Elizabeth was quite the "thinnest looking child I've ever seen" and was shocked even though she knew the girl was diabetic. Anna might have been inclined to be kind to Elizabeth. Not only were their mothers friendly, but Anna also had been very ill the previous summer. She had suffered from a blockage of the mesenteric artery that supplies blood to the intestines, a condition that almost killed her. But if this made Anna empathetic now, she kept it to herself. As a general rule, she did not care to be around children. After one particularly trying afternoon spent with some other American children in town, she dreaded meeting more. "If I have to be nice to children like that all winter, I'll die," she confided to her diary. She found Elizabeth to be different, very "old for her age & quite bright." That gave them something else in common, as Anna saw herself the same way. But Anna was honest enough to admit that, even though she herself was intelligent, her brain "never suffered from overuse." She preferred to spend her time dancing and playing bridge than doing anything else. She and Elizabeth did not warm to each other.

Elizabeth's visiting problems did not last long. Many of her parents' friends such as the Hamlins were there for only a month or two around Christmas, and as they headed back to Washington, this flurry of activity died down. She had to admit that she would miss some of them, especially Mrs. Hamlin, who she found "much the best of all your friends down here." In fact she went so far as to concede that Mrs. Hamlin reminded her of her beloved Mme. Homer, but that was the only compliment she would pay.

Elizabeth hardly retreated into isolation. There were still some people around for her to visit who, like she, were there for the season. She attended meetings of the Girl Guides (the British Girl Scouts) to get to know some girls her own age and went out to enjoy the sights of the island. Between this activity, writing, reading, and needlework, she took her mind off her continuous hunger and her homesickness. Yet as she kept herself occupied, and steadily weakened, something surprising happened. She came into her own.

AWAY FROM HER parents' orbit, and as family friends drifted home, Elizabeth became more confident. Her relationship with Mrs. Burgess changed. The two arranged their days as they wanted, adopted "the cutest tiger kitten you ever knew," and, despite Elizabeth's complaints about the time-consuming demands of visiting, headed out to enjoy the island whenever they felt like it and the weather permitted. With Mrs. Burgess's help, Elizabeth took on some adult responsibilities. Mrs. Hughes had given them an allowance for their discretionary expenses and it was up to them how to use it. Hiring carriages was one of these, but Elizabeth also had to buy her own clothes, and, with Mrs. Burgess, supervise the maid who kept house and cooked for them.

Elizabeth and Mrs. Burgess settled into a companionable relationship. Previously, Elizabeth had addressed her formally. From Lake George, she had written that "Mrs. B. thinks . . ." when explaining something. In Bermuda, she started calling her nurse by her first name, Blanche, and now wrote that "we decided" or "we think" when reporting considering an activity or a change in her diet.

Blanche was no longer the disciplinarian or the only expert on Elizabeth's body. Elizabeth herself had become a partner in her care. When she showed traces of sugar in her urine following the opening of the Washington Conference, she had to reduce her food intake. On the days she traveled to Bermuda, the excitement caused her to have to cut back again. As she settled into Honeymoon Cottage and embarked on her visiting, the two agreed that she needed a few days of eating only 400 calories before settling back into an average of about 700 calories a day.

She and Blanche worked as a team, adjusting her diet so that she quickly managed to get back to 800 calories. And, if Bermuda really worked its soothing magic, they thought she might even be able to increase it beyond that level. "[W]e're slowly increasing my carbohydrate," Elizabeth proudly told her mother. She was bored eating the same thing day after day, so she and Blanche added some celery and spinach. She was pleased "not having touched a thing like that for a year" and she was now "having a wonderful time" with these small variations.

Doctors Frederick Allen and Elliott Joslin would have been pleased. One of the benefits of Allen's treatment plan, apart from prolonging life and easing physical distress, was that it gave patients a sense of control over their lives and allowed them to participate actively in their care. In Bermuda, Elizabeth responded to the diet exactly as they hoped she would.

It was just as well that Elizabeth was feeling more confident because, in this foreign land, she was also her father's representative and had to rise to some international diplomacy, sick as she was. Two particular men, the British governor general, Sir James Willcocks, and Colonel Albert Swalm, the U.S. consul in Bermuda, were not going to leave the daughter of such a powerful man unattended. At first she saw her visits with them as a duty, as they probably did too. However, unlike the routine visits to her mother's friends, she quickly came to enjoy her encounters with them and greatly appreciated their kindness. They became two of the most important relationships she would form in Bermuda.

Of course, Willcocks had pressing professional reasons for wanting to be kind to Secretary Hughes's daughter. The Washington Conference had made the front pages of the

Bermudian paper, the *Royal Gazette,* which had hailed Hughes's proposal for arms limitation as a "masterstroke of open diplomacy." Since Bermuda was an important British military garrison, anything that affected the strategic interests of the Empire got Willcocks's attention. There had also been rumors in the American papers that the United States might buy the Bermudas "with some money owed by Great Britain," a possibility that many of the island's residents found shocking.

Willcocks was an early caller at Honeymoon Cottage. Elizabeth told her mother that he unexpectedly "blew in" on them "just to see how we were getting along, and how we liked Bermuda. I was so overcome, I know I made a fool of myself." Willcocks ignored any awkwardness on Elizabeth's side. "He's a peach," she reported, "I do like him so much!" The feeling was mutual, and he extended invitations to Elizabeth and Blanche for a variety of events at the governor's mansion. Colonel Swalm was, not surprisingly, even more attentive, as this was his boss's daughter, and he may have been acting at the request of Mr. Hughes. Whatever his reasons, he was a thoughtful and generous visitor. Elizabeth was grateful for the care and attention of both men.

Her pleasure in their company was genuine. They were like characters from her books come to life. Colonel Swalm was a spry 86-year-old. He had fought in the Civil War and afterward had a career that had taken him into the American West and South America. He had been a diplomat in Montevideo, Uruguay, for many years, and during that time he and his wife had traveled and had many adventures. Elizabeth excitedly told her mother that on one occasion they had almost lost "their lives crossing the Andes on mule-back in a storm." With stories like that, "you can see why I like to have them call." Visits from Washington society ladies paled in comparison.

James Willcocks could hold his own with this competition. Even though he was a generation younger than Swalm, he had been a lieutenant general in the British Army, serving in Africa and India before commanding a regiment of Indian troops on the Western Front in the recent world war. So both men could feed her appetite for news of distant lands. She had something to offer them, too, apart from being a conduit to her father. She was an attentive, knowledgeable, and eager listener for any stories of their lives they wanted to tell. It was a winning combination.

They were both also considerate about her diet. On one occasion, Elizabeth went to a social event in Hamilton where she unexpectedly found herself seated at an extravagant formal tea. There were no Hoopeses, Hydes, or Homers to joke with. She was trapped beside a table weighed down with food: "endless different kinds of fancy-shaped sandwiches," strawberries and vanilla ice cream, "4 kinds of huge layer cakes, chocolate, date, fruit . . . , plus some cup cakes." Elizabeth wrote that she was "shocked, grieved or surprised when I saw what those poor people were expected to eat"—and what she had to sit next to for much of the afternoon.

Both men immediately recognized her confusion. She later told her mother about it. "I sat completely overwhelmed and had a fine time watching [the other guests] eat . . . . it being the 1st thing of the kind I had ever done or attended, and it put me in a rather unique position." Swalm, sitting next to her, joked that "he'd eat all my shares of everything." But Elizabeth was not the only guest to eat nothing. Willcocks, who sat across from her, did not either. "The sensible Gov. Gen. only took 1 cup of tea the way I did. You know that man only eats dinner & a cup of tea, always omitting his lunch and breakfast." It was an event where she had no control but that good manners committed her to enduring. The two men, especially Willcocks, who Elizabeth thought on this occasion was "more fun than a picnic," made it bearable.

AS JANUARY PASSED, Bermudian winter rains eased and sun returned. Elizabeth and Blanche went out to enjoy the sights of the islands. One day Elizabeth was at the shore, looking out at "the most beautiful scene I have ever seen." They had finished their picnic lunch, and Elizabeth picked up her pen and paper to write a letter to her mother. She began it but found it was "terribly hard to write with such a view and coloring as there is in front of me now and I just sit half the time staring at it!" But write she did.

As she settled into the routine of life in Bermuda, letter writing occupied her mind without using much energy and made her feel connected to her mother and home. Elizabeth wrote every few days, frequently keeping a letter open for a day or two to see if one arrived from her mother containing something she should respond to right away.

Their correspondence was a lifeline for them both. Staying in touch by telephone was not an option. Telephone service, invented in the 1870s, was widely available in much of the United States and Bermuda, but long-distance calls were so expensive and voice transmission of such poor quality that Elizabeth had never even called home from Lake George. Calling her parents from Bermuda was not an option. There was no phone cable between Bermuda and North America, so the phone in her cottage was only for local calls. She could send a telegram in an emergency, but letters were the way she and her mother stayed in touch.

Elizabeth eagerly awaited each of her mother's "lovely letters," looking forward to the arrival of the ships from New York, which all carried any mail that was delivered to them by six A.M. on the day of sailing. Elizabeth eagerly tracked the shipping news in the *Royal Gazette* to know as soon as possible when one had arrived. When there was no letter for her, she was "terribly, terribly disappointed."

In the Hughes household family correspondence was a woman's task, and Mrs. Hughes was the main conduit of information about the whole family. She always made time to write to Elizabeth no matter how relentless her social schedule. Not only were there the ongoing conference activities and what the *Washington Post* described as the "brilliant supper parties" of the holiday season, but the Hugheses had also revived the New Year's Day breakfast for the diplomatic community traditionally hosted by the secretary of state and his wife. So, January 1, 1922, found Mr. and Mrs. Hughes again in the Pan American Union building, meeting and greeting several hundred guests in a flag-draped Hall of the Americas. Mrs. Hughes could not look forward to a relaxing afternoon. All the cabinet wives were scheduled to be "at home" for visitors so New Year's wishes could be exchanged.

There was no letup in the following weeks. Mrs. Hughes was a "patroness" for a fundraising ball for the Columbia Hospital for Women. That was followed shortly thereafter by a "brilliant reception" President and Mrs. Harding hosted for the Supreme Court justices. According to the *Post,* Antoinette looked lovely in a gown of "rose velvet made with a long train and a surplice waist." Despite these events, other obligations, and many sessions with her dressmaker, Mrs. Hughes regularly sat down to write long, newsy letters to Elizabeth.

Elizabeth had no expectation that her father would find time to write to her. Nor did she look for any letter from her brother, Charlie. He had sent her five dollars for Christmas (a generous sum in 1921) and she wrote and thanked him. Otherwise, Mrs. Hughes forwarded his news and, on one occasion, a letter from him, which Elizabeth returned to her mother after she had read.

Elizabeth did expect her sister Catherine to correspond occasionally. When she traveled in Europe after graduating from Wellesley, Catherine sent Elizabeth postcards. But once she was back in the United States, moving between her brother in New York and her parents' home in Washington, it was Mrs. Hughes who usually passed on her news. Catherine did occasionally pen a letter and Elizabeth wrote in response, enclosing the letter in the envelope with the one for her mother.

Letters are usually private communications, but they can involve communities of writers and readers. Elizabeth frequently wrote her letters in Blanche's company and chatted while she did so. Occasionally, she relayed a message from Blanche or Blanche herself added a postscript. Although

Mrs. Hughes was the recipient, she shared their contents if not the letters themselves with others, so Elizabeth knew her news would be passed on to the whole family.

She was already a skilled letter writer. She had learned the conventions of letter writing at school and home, and that was bolstered by advice in the children's magazines to which she subscribed, especially the weekly *Youth's Companion*. It encouraged its readers to see a well-written letter as an artistic creation that required the same thought and effort they would put into any other. It also wisely recommended that a writer not mail a letter as soon as it was written. Rather, it should be kept unsealed overnight to be read again in the morning to make sure that it did not contain "any personal remark . . . that might cause pain or mischief if seen by anyone for whom the letter was not meant."

Elizabeth's mother gave her advice, too, and had trained her to write prompt thank-you letters. When she was younger, her mother looked over them to make sure they were correct. Even now that she was older, when Elizabeth wrote a formal thank-you to people she did not know well, she wished her mother's "eagle eye had run over it" to save her from embarrassing mistakes.

Even though her letters were sometimes written over several days, almost as a journal, Elizabeth never departed from the conventions. Beginning with "Dear Mumsey," her writing was warm and playful. She wrote as if she were speaking and signed off with lots of affectionate wishes ("more love than words can ever express") and the simple signature "Me!!" She felt comfortable writing both formally and with slang. Great

One of Elizabeth's letters to her mother. Courtesy the Thomas Fisher Rare Book Library, University of Toronto.

days were "corking," and enjoyable events or particularly nice people were "peachy." Her letters were filled with exclamation marks and dashes that gave emphasis to her writing.

The conversational tone of Elizabeth's letters may have come naturally to her, but it was also recommended by *Youth's Companion*. The magazine encouraged its readers to think of themselves as having a conversation with the people to whom they were writing. That way, they could express themselves with "freedom from artificiality, [and with] the cheerfulness and the grace and humor of conversation."

Elizabeth saw the primary function of her letters as imparting news of her daily activities, and she wrote even when "[n]othing much has happened except for the ordinary things of life." She included her thoughts about others. A Bermudian girl her own age, Caroline Cooper, was "sweet," and new acquaintances of her parents' age were "charming people." When a friend of her parents in Bermuda, Miss Parmalee, postponed an excursion in which Elizabeth had been included because it was raining, Elizabeth moaned that it was "just like her." Her letters, though, were mostly an upbeat recounting of her days. After the excursion with Miss Parmalee was canceled, for example, she and Blanche took themselves out anyway, as they had ordered a carriage and both thoroughly enjoyed their drive along the South Shore, where "the surf was marvelous" to watch.

Writing letters offered Elizabeth a distraction from her hunger. For both her and her mother, the correspondence also provided a comforting emotional connection and reassured them that Elizabeth was leading something like a normal life. When people write about themselves, they choose what aspect of their lives is important to mention. Elizabeth's letters could have reflected the intense focus on her body that her illness required. After all, chronic illness profoundly alters one's identity and experience and even though Elizabeth did not know she was dying, diabetes had changed her life forever. But she rarely mentioned it either directly or indirectly.

Part of the reason for this was the continuing mutual pretense in which she and her mother were engaged, each creating for the other a sense that everything was still as it had ever been. But there was also a practical reason. Her letters were reporting the news, and her illness was not news. Also, it was not one that caused specific pain that could be reported; rather, she would have felt generally very weak. There was little new to say about it.

She might have been writing cheerful letters because that was what she wanted to receive—letters that would cheer her up, help her through her illness, and keep her engaged with the world. She was also describing her life to people she cared about and who worried about her. She presented the familiar daughter as a way of comforting her parents and, perhaps, herself. Portraying herself as the jaunty, engaged, social Elizabeth was not false. It was just not the whole story.

But it was the way she chose to present herself. She kept her letters focused on the positive and downplayed the inconveniences of her condition. She mentioned it only when, for example, she described the changes that she and Blanche were making to her diet, or when on a trip to the dressmaker she chose an extra-wide piece of lace on a collar because without it she looked "too much like myself, narrow and scrimpy." Otherwise, it was Bermuda and "the ordinary things of life" that featured in her letters.

It is also possible that with her upbeat tone she was just

trying to think positively. Theories of the power of positive thinking, autosuggestion, had appeared in 1909. Its supporters believed that physical and mental problems could be overcome by the conscious mind making an extra effort to make the "repair of some deficiency." Although this theory would not peak in popularity until the 1920s, when the writings of the French psychotherapist Émile Coué were translated, ideas about autosuggestion circulated widely long before then.

Elizabeth's strict adherence to the correct letter-writing form suggests another reason for keeping her letters upbeat: it was simply unmannerly to write about sad things. Emily Post, the most important etiquette writer of the day, admonished that there was no excuse for writers to put "all their troubles and fears of troubles out on paper" and write "needlessly of misfortune or unhappiness." Doing so simply created heartache for the recipient, and Elizabeth did not want to do that.

On one occasion in early January, though, Elizabeth had to confront her illness as openly as she ever did in a letter after her mother told her some exciting family news. Catherine had become engaged to Chauncey Waddell and the wedding would be in June. Elizabeth thought it "most thrilling." Her mother also told her that Catherine and Chauncey wanted her to be a maid of honor, but Catherine and Mrs. Hughes thought it would be too much for her and had decided against it. Thus, the offer was extended and withdrawn at the same time. Elizabeth was gracious. "I understand perfectly all about the Maid of Honor business," she told her mother, "much the wisest plan." For the next two full pages of her letter, she tried to convince herself of this. "I get . . . without knowing it terribly upset inside over those things and a good share of the benefit of my being down here might be upset completely you know.... That kind of thing always affects me so easily," she opined. "It would be almost better for me to be an 'interested onlooker'... [and] I don't really want to leave before June anyway." She asked her mother to "Tell [Catherine] how much I appreciate her's and Chauncey's wanting me and all." None of this sounded very convincing.

But her mother's next letter in mid-January brought news that took Elizabeth's mind off any disappointment she felt about the wedding. The end of the Washington Conference seemed to be in sight, and Mr. Hughes could clear his calendar for them to visit Bermuda at the end of the month. Elizabeth was "too happy and excited for words."

There was suddenly a lot to do, getting extra linens for Honeymoon Cottage, coming up with a list of things for her mother to bring, offering her clothing advice ("a great many hats are not necessary, although you want plenty of course"), and planning sightseeing trips. The Hugheses' imminent visit was quickly public knowledge. When Elizabeth heard that people were already planning public events, she made Colonel Swalm promise to "protect" them as much as possible.

Elizabeth tried to wait patiently. She settled into a routine that allowed her to conserve her energy, getting up late and taking a rest after lunch. She did a little visiting and attended Girl Guide meetings. There, she joined the other girls in planning a fundraising bazaar for early February. She was very pleased when her new guide friend, Caroline, asked her to sell at her table. Elizabeth got busy stitching small items to sell and, recognizing her own lack of skill ("you know I'm not a born sewer"), asked her mother to buy her badly made items when she came to the event. She eagerly looked forward to hearing when her parents' ship would arrive.

JANUARY 1922 ALSO proved to be an interesting time for the young chemist Bert Collip, who had now joined the Toronto research team. In fact, it turned out to be one of the most dramatic months of his life. The work he was doing on the extract was, he told Henry Tory, his boss back at the University of Alberta, "an absolutely satisfactory experience," thrilling even. His task was to take the "mysterious something" that had been extracted from animal pancreases and that seemed to work effectively in dogs and render it in "a form suitable for human administration." It was a daunting challenge but, even if he was unsuccessful, he would still have been part of a milestone "in the field of carbohydrate metabolism."

While he was working on this, his family life was causing him lots of anxiety. His wife, Ray, was at home with their two young daughters, and the second child, Barbara, only a few months old, was very ill. In her short life, she had already had diphtheria and pneumonia. Now everyone in the household except him had contracted influenza. Ray's sister came to stay to nurse everyone but she, too, fell ill. Collip did not want to get sick himself and so stayed at the lab 24 hours a day. Whatever Ray felt about this, it meant that Collip could work on his project every waking moment.

The other researchers were on similar professional and personal roller-coaster rides. At the end of December, Banting,

Best, Collip, and Macleod had gone to Yale University to present their results to the American Physiological Society. In the audience to hear the talk were Frederick Allen, Elliott Joslin, Israel Kleiner, and other luminaries of diabetic research. They were a tough audience and needed convincing that the group had done more than others who had achieved promising results only to see even worse side effects.

Banting made his presentation awkwardly and then faced challenging questions. The experiments had not been as rigorous as they might have been. The scientists were concerned that the Toronto group had not done some obvious things. For example, fever had been a common side effect of earlier extracts, yet Banting and Best had not thought to take the dogs' temperatures. Macleod, watching his junior colleague struggling, stepped in to defend the team's work. He asserted their positive accomplishments in his usual assured way. Macleod was pleased to save the day, but Banting saw the professor as usurping his role and was furious. In the days that followed, Banting began to speak openly to his friends at the lab that Macleod was trying to steal his work.

Despite that drama and the generally cautious reception to the research, there was someone in the audience who was very interested in the group's findings: George Clowes of Eli Lilly & Company. In 1920, Clowes had become director of research for Lilly and was a skilled chemist in his own right. Born in England, he had attended a number of prestigious European universities, finally earning his PhD from Göttingen University in Germany. His primary research interest was in cancer, and he had worked for many years at the Institute for Malignant

Diseases in Buffalo, New York. He had been hired by Lilly as part of a bold innovation in which the company created its own research arm that worked closely with academic and other scientists. Clowes saw potential in the new extract and offered his company's services to Banting and Macleod when they were ready to make it commercially.

They were still a long way from that, although Banting was lobbying hard to be allowed to conduct a formal human test. Through the university's relationship with Toronto General Hospital, doctors there chose a boy Elizabeth's age, 14-year-old Leonard Thompson, to receive the first injection of the extract. Leonard had been starving on Allen's plan and had stayed alive for three years but was now near death, consuming only about 450 calories a day. His father consented to Leonard receiving the experimental substance. On January 11, he received a shot but it had little effect. There was only a small reduction in his blood sugar levels and he developed a sterile abscess at the injection site as a result of impurities in the extract. Banting was mortified.

While he came to terms with that disappointment, Bert Collip made two dramatic discoveries. The first was that he discovered, by accident and quick thinking, that the extract had the potential to be fatal. He had given rabbits in his lab an unusually large dose of the extract, and they had convulsed and died. At first he thought there was something wrong with the extract. When another rabbit began to convulse, he quickly took a blood sample and then gave the animal some glucose solution to see what would happen. It recovered. The rabbit had convulsed because the large doses of extract had reduced its blood sugar to extremely low levels. Glucose revived it. Today, this phenomenon is known as insulin shock or hypoglycemic reaction. A graduate student, Oliver Gaebler, who watched these events unfold later recalled that Collip's actions were "the most thinking per square meter per minute that I have ever seen."

Collip's second accomplishment was that he succeeded in rendering the extract "suitable for human administration." He had worked hard, continuously adjusting the many variables, solvents, filtration times and techniques, and the length of time and pace of evaporation, among many others things. When he realized that he had finally done it, he quickly telephoned Ray to tell her the news. A few days later, on January 23, Leonard Thompson received some of Collip's new extract. His blood sugar level quickly dropped to normal. In another letter to Tory in Alberta, Collip told him about this "phenomenal break."

What he did not tell Tory was that no one was popping champagne corks to celebrate. Instead, tempers were flaring again, and this time it was Collip who was at the center of the storm. When the young chemist had gone to tell Banting about his "break," he refused to tell him how he had treated the extract and a fight erupted. Collip may have felt that he was obliged to tell only Macleod the details. Or he might have been afraid that Banting, of an unpredictable temper, would not recognize his contribution publicly. Or it may have been simply a misunderstanding due to exhaustion on all sides. Best later recalled that Banting was so angry that he had to restrain him "with all the force at my command." Clark Noble, a graduate student of Macleod's and a good friend of Best's, some time later drew a cartoon of the argument. It has not survived, but it featured Banting sitting on top of Collip, his hands around Collip's throat, with the caption "The Discovery of Insulin."

Colleagues quickly corralled the four men, Banting, Best, Macleod, and Collip, to defuse the situation and come up with a plan for how they should proceed. The result was a formal document they all signed on January 25 in which they agreed that none of them would try to patent the substance independently of the others. They also committed to working with the university's Connaught Anti-Toxin Laboratories, set up a few years earlier, to develop larger-scale manufacturing of the extract when there was enough clinical evidence to confirm its effectiveness.

Early February was an exciting time. Some additional money and staff became available so that the clinical evidence could be gathered. Collip had assistants to help him make the extract and Macleod and doctors at Toronto General were working on designing studies to examine the physiological responses in the recipients. A few more hospital patients began receiving the extract, as did Banting's friend Joe Gilchrist, and a new round of animal testing also began.

Banting found himself on the sidelines. He had initiated the whole enterprise but now others were in control. He was miserable.

ELIZABETH WAS ON an emotional roller-coaster ride herself as January drew to a close. Things had been looking up. Her parents were due to arrive soon; Blanche had rowed her out in a borrowed boat to explore some small islands; Governor

Willcocks had invited them over to Government House to watch a game of "tent-pegging," similar to polo, and to the Garrison Theatre for a great evening's entertainment, a musical review that the British officers and their families put on called "5,000 Years Ago." Movies or concerts in local halls and hotels were few, so the officers and men made their own entertainment. The *Royal Gazette* hailed this amateur production as "the most elaborate piece of stage-craft ever seen in Bermuda." Elizabeth thought it was "really wonderful," though she was equally entertained watching what she called the Bermudian "royalty"—the governor general, an admiral, and the chief justice, who all attended.

And she had received a piece of good news. An essay she had submitted to a competition in a children's magazine to which she subscribed, *St. Nicholas,* was awarded a "special mention." The magazine printed only the essays that won gold or silver stars (first and second prizes), but the readers whose essays came third earned a special mention and had the pleasure of seeing their names in print and of knowing that their work "would have been used had space permitted." The magazine invited 300-word submissions from readers in response to a prompt, such as "my favorite holiday." Writing something to submit had been a satisfying task for Elizabeth for some months, and she began to see it as an investment in her future.

She already had enjoyed seeing some of her essays in print. She'd had her first triumph the previous summer. In response to the prompt "a proud moment," she wrote about a family fishing trip on a previous visit to Lake George and her essay was published in the September 1921 issue, winning a silver star. This success filled her with "great veal and zigor" (an old joke), and she afterward regularly sent in short essays. She asked her mother to tell her father that this was "the first step toward his 'life' that I am bound I am going to write some day."

Elizabeth enjoyed the challenge of writing these essays. They needed to be more formal than her letters home and required careful planning, revising, and editing. Typewriters had been invented about 50 years earlier, but they were seen as a business tool and few people had them at home. Without one, Elizabeth had to rewrite her essays neatly when she was ready to submit them. Then, there was always the possibility of rejection and she would not know the results for months. Despite the formality, her essays were entertaining. In the humorous story of the family fishing trip, she related how a hooked trout ended up "entangled, hook and all, in Mother's pretty dress, and commenced flopping in her lap." The brief story required five exclamation marks to tell.

Her hard work paid off. Only two months after her initial success, she won a gold star in the November 1921 *St. Nicholas* for her essay on the topic "my favorite episode in American history." For that assignment, she chose Robert E. Lee's surrender to Ulysses S. Grant at Appomattox Court House in 1865. Grant was, she wrote, "in the height of his glory."

Each publishing success made her even more determined to continue. Competing made her feel connected to "boys and girls all over the country" who were doing the same thing. Anne Homer, one of the Homer twins with whom she had spent a lot of time at Lake George, was one of them. In January, when

Elizabeth's essay received a "special mention," Anne had an essay published and Elizabeth was happy for her.

Writing helped her imagine a future life for herself. She never considered it to be a chore. "How I do love writing," she exclaimed in a letter. Her successes made her feel "that perhaps after all, I may be able to write some day." She was philosophical if an essay was not published, because she thought it was "really lots of fun trying for things." She told her mother "it's my highest ambition to write" but thought she might still be too young to start a serious career, asking, "[W]hen can you begin—I wonder—sending things to magazines? Is it just quality or does age count too?" She saw her essay submissions as training for her future career.

But as January came to an end, Elizabeth faced new challenges. The first was "a terrible disappointment." Her parents had to postpone their visit by a couple of weeks because the Washington Conference was dragging on. The four major world powers, the United States, France, Britain, and Japan, were negotiating an agreement to conclude the conference but the proceedings were held up by Japan's claim to the Shantung region of China. These nations would eventually sign the Four Power Treaty but, in the meantime, Elizabeth had to "hope for the best and curse old Shantung!" She told her mother not to "worry about me pining away" over the delay. Her "adopted policy," she declared, "is 'Expect them when you see them and never look forward to anything too much,'" the words of someone who was, if not pining, clearly disappointed.

As she heard the news of the postponement, she again showed traces of sugar. Fortunately, the next day was her scheduled fast day, a day when she ate only about 320 calories, and so her urine was soon clear. She tried to focus on another event she was looking forward to, the Girl Guide Bazaar on February 11 in Par-la-Ville, a park in the center of Hamilton. This event meant a lot to her. Her family was deeply involved in the scouting movement, even though it was relatively new. The Girl Guides had been organized in Britain as recently as 1910 and in the United States as the Girl Scouts the following year, but Elizabeth's sister Helen had quickly got involved. She had been a troop leader before she died and Catherine still was one. Elizabeth had been a Girl Scout in Washington and already had earned several merit badges before she came to Bermuda. She took her commitment seriously.

She felt her sewing was not enough of a contribution to the event, so she also made candy and put it into little enamel boxes she had painted by hand. Few things stand as a greater testament to her desire to be involved and stay connected to girls her age than her decision to make fudge and butter-scotch the Thursday before the bazaar, a day when she herself ate fewer than 750 calories. She had committed to selling on a flower stall and to offering "miscellaneous items" with her friend at the Saturday event. It was an exhausting day, hardly surprising as she weighed a mere 53 pounds, but she would not have missed it.

Afterward, Elizabeth did not sit down to write to her mother as she often did on Sunday evenings. Her parents were scheduled to arrive imminently. However, at the last moment, they telegraphed that they would be delayed a few more days before they could sail. Elizabeth was sad, but she had found a community in Bermuda and was coming to love the island. Her diet was going well. She had become more confident and her writing success was making her optimistic about future possibilities. Surely things were looking up.

CHAPTER 6

Oh How I Dote on Reading

O N FEBRUARY 17, 1922, the Hugheses made their much anticipated arrival in Bermuda. Hundreds of American tourists and local residents lined the waterfront to greet them. The couple had needed Blanche's remedy for seasickness as the journey, the *Royal Gazette* reported, "was not of the smoothest." That was an understatement. The *New York Times* called it "one of the roughest the steamer Fort Hamilton has ever experienced." Still, Mr. Hughes told those who greeted him that he was delighted with the "service rendered" on board.

All the leaders of the British colonial administration and military garrison were on the dock to welcome them, with Elizabeth and Blanche standing with the governor general, James Willcocks. The *Gazette* reported "a pretty incident" took place as the gangway was put in place. General Willcocks should have walked up it first as the highest-ranking person present, but he was too good a man to stand on such ceremony. He "bade Miss Hughes lead the way up the gangway so that she might be the first to greet her father," which she did. Colonel Albert Swalm, the U.S. consul, then made the formal introductions. The governor kindly made his carriage available so the entire Hughes party could make their way to Honeymoon Cottage once the brief welcoming ceremony was over. Then, Elizabeth and her parents settled in for a long chat to catch up.

Colonel Swalm did his best to protect the Hugheses' time. He had promised Elizabeth he would, and even the *Gazette* reminded its readers that the couple's visit was private. Still, several events were unavoidable. They made a courtesy visit to Governor and Mrs. Willcocks at Government House shortly after their arrival, and later the Willcockses hosted an informal dinner for them. But the Hugheses were not going to get out of official activities so lightly. Even though Mr. Hughes himself reminded people that this was a private visit, the Bermuda Trade Development Board convinced him that "Bermuda would feel grieved" if he did not make himself available. Thus, the board hosted an afternoon reception at the Princess Hotel in Hamilton at which 500 guests had the pleasure of meeting the pair. The *Gazette* declined to list the attendees individually but simply noted that "everyone who could possibly be there was there."

Despite these events, and a tree-planting ceremony on the day before their departure, it was, Elizabeth thought, "a satisfactory and lovely, lovely visit," and she pined for them when they left. Her mother thoughtfully did not make her wait days for her next letter. She sent one back by the pilot boat that escorted their ship into open water, and Elizabeth told her that it "comforted me a great deal."

Her parents had been worried when they saw her. Despite all the upbeat reports Elizabeth had sent, she was frail. They thought she had been trying to do too much and so bought a hammock for the garden to encourage her to stay home. In early March, just before her parents left, she developed an eye infection and a cough that kept her awake at night for a long time afterward. Even so, she was reluctant to stay home and rest. "I am curbing myself . . . although it goes against my poor 'ambish' [ambition] most terribly." But she did recognize that she was weaker. She joked with her mother it was just as well she was "going to be a writer, for they don't have to use their legs! Te He!" It was hollow humor.

Now that her mother was back in Washington, Elizabeth insisted that her diet was going well, that she was gaining slowly in strength, and that "[e]verybody says I'm looking better." But they were just being nice. After she recovered from her cough, she had a bad fall in the cottage, breaking her glasses, cutting her face, and getting a fragment of glass in her eye. Fortunately, Blanche was able to get it out quickly, but Elizabeth bemoaned the fact that as soon as she had "fully recovered from one thing, something else seems to happen." She had tripped on the rug while carrying their supper dishes from the kitchen to the dining room. It was not food that she was going to eat, though; she was carrying bread and bacon for Blanche.

Weakening and spending more and more time in the garden hammock without complaint, Elizabeth turned for escape into the world of books. Reading not only passed the time and took her mind off her lack of energy; it also liberated her from the dehumanizing and regimenting nature of Allen's plan, the necessity to monitor her body's processes, record every morsel of food eaten, take multiple daily urine tests, and observe her body's general response to her diet. As the Bermudian spring passed, she spent many hours lost in a good book.

READING OFFERED HER an unadulterated pleasure. The essay writing she did had the potential for disappointment, and visiting was tiring and came with the tension of being around food, but a good book offered complete escape. "Oh how I dote on reading," she exclaimed in a letter to her mother. Elizabeth read voraciously, and her letters home from this time were filled with details of what book was in her hands, what she had finished, and what she thought she might read next. One choice, she declared, was "the most interesting book." It was by the nature and travel writer William Henry Hudson, and was about his early life living on the pampas of Argentina. "[W]ith such beautiful descriptions of that wild ranch life," she reported, "no wonder I enjoyed it immensely."

Elizabeth loved natural history and travel writing, and Hudson was her favorite author. She occasionally chose a work of fiction, but only when it featured an interesting location or vivid descriptions of the natural world. It was most commonly a work of Hudson's that lay on her lap. His books are little read today. His long, flowery sentences, the slow pace of his travel, and his quiet contemplation of the landscape have gone out of fashion.

However, Elizabeth loved his style and copied it when she wanted to describe scenic beauty. "Oh the brightness of this moon as it shone," she exclaimed after an evening picnic. They had eaten by the "light of a most gorgeous sunset, that filled whole heaven with a pink glow, in which rose our white moon sending its bright rays over the now comparatively tranquil and peaceful sea. Oh it was an unforgettable scene!" Elizabeth had perhaps been reading too much Hudson!

She read other nature writers but in Hudson, she found a kindred spirit. Like her, he had little opportunity for formal education and was not able to be physically active. At about Elizabeth's age, he had suffered from typhus and rheumatic fever and as an adult, he was badly injured in an accident. Consequently, his books were not taken up in the details of travel; rather, he wrote as a static observer of the world around him. Born in 1841 on a ranch in Argentina to American parents, Hudson focused many of his books on his childhood there and his journeys around Latin America. In his writings, he blended a spiritual and inspirational appreciation of nature with meticulous scientific observation. His work enjoyed a large following on both sides of the Atlantic, and Elizabeth was delighted to find that the library in Hamilton was well supplied with Hudson titles. His work was so popular there that the *Gazette* made a point of mentioning it on page one when the library acquired his latest book.

Elizabeth made regular use of that library. When she was at Lake George, she read Mrs. Hoopes's books and some she had brought with her. In Bermuda, the rental cottage had little to offer her and she had been able to bring only one or two of her own books on the voyage. The Hamilton library supplied her needs. There was a tiny bookstore, too, but Elizabeth was on a tight budget. The library was only in two large rooms, but it had benefited from the attentive care of a single administrator for 40 years and its collection was rich. Seasonal visitors could check books out for just a few pennies. Elizabeth found her tastes well supplied in this corner of the empire.

It is not surprising that Elizabeth loved reading. She had grown up in a household in which books were revered. When her father was a child, he always had his nose in a book. Although he occasionally read fiction, such as Daniel Defoe's 18th-century novel *Robinson Crusoe,* he preferred nonfiction such as Charles Coffin's 1870 travel narrative *The Seat of Empire.* He loved its vivid descriptions of the "vast reach of country lying between the [great] lakes and the Pacific in the United States and British America [Canada]."

As a young boy and into his adult life, Hughes loved both to travel and to read about the journeys of others. As an only child, his favorite game had been "travel," in which he rode his hobby horse in his attic playroom to imaginary parts of the world, sometimes with a book open on the floor in front of him to consult about what he would be "seeing." Part of the appeal of the game was that he could escape his highly disciplined home life. The people he read about in Coffin's book had escaped, too. They had "cut loose from all care, and enjoyed a few weeks of freedom and recreation" in the American Northwest.

As an adult, Hughes chose to do the same. When he came close to collapsing from overwork, he set off for the mountains. He shared the feelings of the Scottish naturalist John Muir that mountains offered rejuvenation. Muir wrote, "Come to the mountains and get their good tidings." Hughes went and got them. He traveled alone to Europe to climb in the Swiss Alps.

On his return, he again turned to travel literature and enjoyed Amelia Edwards's *Untrodden Peaks and Unfrequented Valleys,* about the Dolomites in Italy, so much that he promptly made plans to go there the following year.

Mrs. Hughes read avidly too, a solace that had helped her through her lonely childhood. It was a pleasure that continued into her adult life, and as she went off to Wellesley, a women's college, she read broadly. She was lucky to have the opportunity to go. At the time, the 1880s, less than 4 percent of Americans went to college, and women made up less than 20 percent of even that small number. College curricula involved more memorization than critical thinking, and so personal reading was a primary part of the intellectual journey. Students got together informally to discuss the books they read. But what one read was also an indicator of social status and education, so Antoinette had to choose carefully what she would read—or at least what she was going to talk about and be seen reading. Her love of books stayed with her after she married and raised her children.

Elizabeth, then, grew up in a family with a love of travel and reading. Unfortunately for her, they had done most of their overseas excursions before she was born and her father became a public figure. When her brother, Charlie, was 12, he was allowed to accompany his father on a European tour and three years later, in 1905, two years before Elizabeth was born, the Hugheses took all three of their children to Europe. After her father's career took off, there was rarely the opportunity for him to indulge his own or his family's inclinations for foreign travel. Instead they vacationed in Maine, at Lake George, or out on Long Island.

But why might she not be able to see distant lands in the future? Her sojourn in Bermuda had already opened up a world to her that she had never expected. For the moment, though, she was content experiencing the larger world as her father had in his attic as a child, through books and her imagination. Fortunately, she had a good supply of both.

As she languished in the hammock, Elizabeth's choice of reading was decidedly grown up. She rarely read books directed to her age group. One would expect, at 14, her reading choices to be driven by pleasure in a good story, and she did read some short stories and serials in magazines. But she more generally eschewed fiction and told her parents that she preferred the "reading of good books not silly novels and baby stories that don't do you any good and that you forget immediately." She may have been just reflecting her father's sentiment here and repeated it to please him, but she could not have devoured nonfiction books at the pace she did if they had not captivated her. When she read yet another Hudson book, for example, she invariably noted it with exclamation points or underlining: "I just love him!"

She also followed her parents' habit of reading the newspapers assiduously. While she was in Bermuda, in addition to the *Royal Gazette,* Elizabeth subscribed to the *Washington Post* and the *Herald,* to follow her father's activities and other world and local events. These papers did not arrive daily but came in bundles on the steamships that docked two or three times a week.

This reading also helped her to know something about the people she met in Bermuda. She encountered Norman Irving

Black, an American painter who divided his time between Bermuda and Maine. He gave her a gift of one of his works, which she greatly appreciated. She also met Augusta Rosenwald, the wife of Julius Rosenwald, the president of the Sears Roebuck Corporation and a self-made man. He had become one of the country's richest men and the couple among its most famous philanthropists, giving away tens of millions of dollars. Mrs. Rosenwald had a great interest in children's issues. She gave money to the Juvenile Protective Association, an organization that worked to shape public policy on child welfare issues, and was an honorary vice president of the American Girl Scouts.

Mr. and Mrs. Hughes had met Mrs. Rosenwald during their stay in Bermuda. Later, Elizabeth also met her when, because of her interest in scouting, she had lunch with a small group of Girl Guides. Elizabeth enjoyed seeing her. They did not meet again but before Mrs. Rosenwald left for New York, she gave Elizabeth a present of a soft wool blanket to use in the garden hammock. "Wasn't it perfectly lovely and nice" of her, Elizabeth exclaimed. She was delighted by the gift and enjoyed using it whenever she settled down to read.

Though Elizabeth's taste in reading was mature, by age she was an adolescent, not a developmental category into which she easily fit. The term "adolescence" had only recently been coined at about the time of her brother's teen years. The Harvard psychologist G. Stanley Hall had published a book entitled *Adolescence* in 1904. Hall popularized a view of adolescence as a distinct period during which young people experienced great emotional upheaval that required specific institutions and activities to navigate, and his ideas had quickly gained wide currency. That life stage was usually defined by school grade, but Elizabeth had not attended school for several years and had limited contact with children her own age. She did not feel bound by the demarcation lines of the educational system, nor was she influenced much by the reading choices of other children.

Despite her mature tastes and interests, she was still physically immature. She had not gone through puberty. Ever since she was 11 years old, her body had been starved of nourishment. Good nutrition and healthy height–weight ratios are critical for the onset of menarche in girls and sexual development in general. Additionally, undernutrition and falling between 10 and 15 percent below normal weight for height causes amenorrhea (cessation of periods) if menarche has already begun. Stress also delays the onset of puberty. For multiple reasons, then, Elizabeth's physical development could not continue after her diagnosis. So she stayed in a child's body but matured emotionally and intellectually.

The only reading contact she maintained with the world of childhood was children's magazines. The monthly to which she submitted essays, *St. Nicholas,* was her particular favorite. She loved its mostly serialized adventure stories. These involved self-confident young people, functioning without too much grown-up supervision, who solved mysteries or tackled difficult life circumstances with determination and daring. The magazine also had regular math puzzles and a section that summarized national and international news. Elizabeth eagerly awaited each issue that her mother forwarded from Washington.

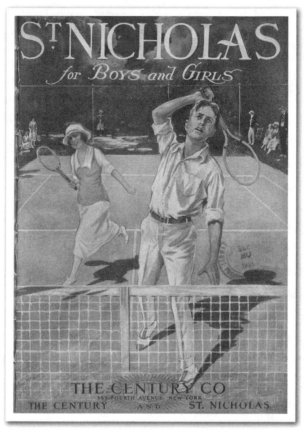

St. Nicholas, *September 1921. Courtesy Library of Congress.*

She also received *American Girl, Every Land,* and *Youth's Companion.* The first was the magazine of the American Girl Scouts. *Every Land* promoted Christian missionary activity. Elizabeth never learned who had arranged its subscription, but she enjoyed it for its reports from missionaries with "interesting stories of China, India, Japan etc." The weekly *Youth's Companion* was one of the most popular children's magazines of the period. After the Civil War, a new owner, Daniel Sharp Ford, pitched it at children but included reading for the whole family. It was filled with stories, puzzles, and a digest of news and other information such as etiquette tips and suitable party treats. Ford's stable of writers had to submit stories with good plots, "at least one strong incident," but no bad language or "evil passions." He also insisted that there be no religious, political, sectional, or class bias to ensure that the magazine have the broadest market appeal. At its peak in the 1890s, the weekly magazine sold more than 500,000 copies, although its circulation was in decline by the time Elizabeth was a reader.

Elizabeth loved this breadth of content. Apart from *American Girl,* she read no magazines directed specifically at her despite the fact that, years earlier, marketers had identified middle- and upper-class girls with allowances in their pockets as an important market and created magazines for them. Instead, Elizabeth preferred the general adventure stories that featured boys and girls, the puzzles, and world news in *St. Nicholas* and *Youth's Companion* and, in the case of *Every Land,* the locations.

St. Nicholas was not the only magazine to which she submitted essays; she had also sent one to *Every Land* entitled "Our North American Indians." It, too, was published, and her prize was a book chosen from the magazine's approved list. She selected an account of the work of the Scottish missionary David Livingstone in Africa, probably reflecting her interest in travel and adventure as much as religion. Elizabeth rarely entered a church, never mentioned praying, and never celebrated her delight in nature in anything but secular terms. Her family was a member of Calvary Baptist Church on 8th and H streets in Washington but did not attend regularly. Elizabeth had gone to church once or twice at Lake George, but there was no Baptist church in Bermuda and she attended no other services.

Her lack of religious reading or activity is striking for a girl who was the granddaughter of a Baptist minister and whose father was, while governor of New York, president of the Northern Baptist Convention. However, he had long since stepped back from what he called "formal religious observances." Charles Evan Hughes was a man of profound faith but felt that it "transcended the narrow limits of our church creeds." Elizabeth followed her family into the church but otherwise made no reference to religious beliefs. They were not part of her correspondence, her activities, or, apart from *Every Land* and her book on Livingstone, her reading.

She did not read or reread some of the classic children's books of the era that showed readers ways of coping with the challenges of suffering. Through the tragic portrayal of the dying Little Eva in the best-selling *Uncle Tom's Cabin* and the noble suffering of Beth March in *Little Women* and Katy in *What Katy Did,* readers were taught how to conduct themselves in the face of chronic illness and grief. However, Elizabeth in her own crisis did not turn to these books for solace, guidance, or entertainment. Elizabeth read for escape.

Yet, surprisingly, she did not look for escape reading or rereading adventure stories. There were plenty of these to choose from, including Laura Lee Hope's *The Bobbsey Twins,* who had made their debut in 1913; Lucy Maud Montgomery's *Anne of Green Gables;* and Anna Sewall's *Black Beauty.* Francis

Hodgson Burnett's *The Secret Garden* would have been a logical choice too, especially as Burnett was in Bermuda at the same time as Elizabeth. All these classics sparked readers' imaginations. They featured resourceful heroines who solved problems, rose above inappropriate anger or envy, and dealt nobly with the challenges that were thrown at them.

But Elizabeth had left behind whatever pleasures she might have found in these books. They were not what she leaned on now when she wanted escape, empowerment, solace, or to suppress her anger at the hand fate had dealt her. Instead, she wanted to read about the world that she hoped she would one day see. She wanted to experience vicariously the delights of places described by Hudson and others. She wanted to lose herself not in a story of adventure or consolation but in accounts of distant lands that were, according to Hudson, "soul-satisfying."

AS ELIZABETH READ in her hammock, the Hughes household back in Washington was a hive of activity. Catherine's engagement had been publicly announced a few days after her parents returned from their trip, setting the wheels in motion for a huge society wedding. It had been decided during the Hugheses' visit to Bermuda that Elizabeth and Blanche would not even attend the wedding that was now set for June 10, 1922. The two would stay in Bermuda until after all the chaos and excitement had passed. Elizabeth had thought her parents might use Greystone for the reception, but she had not realized the scale of the event. Instead, by early April they had settled on the Pan American Union, a building with which the

Hugheses were quite familiar. They would need the space. The guests numbered in the thousands.

Now, it was Elizabeth's turn to be worried about her parents and Catherine. She was sure they were all "tearing their hair in every direction!" over the wedding plans. But she was especially concerned about her mother. "Please don't get all worn out through it all, Mumsey," she wrote. Mrs. Hughes had little choice. She had three months to prepare. With a guest list that included President and Mrs. Harding, Vice President and Mrs. Coolidge, the entire cabinet and spouses, ditto the Supreme Court justices, and what seemed to be the entire diplomatic corps, not to mention family and friends, neither Mrs. Hughes nor Catherine was going to be resting anytime soon.

Despite this compassion, Elizabeth gave her mother a few additional chores. She asked her to send some money to an orphan she had "adopted" in France; had her renew her subscription to her *American Girl* magazine; and asked her for another favor. A Mrs. Noyes, a friend of her mother's, had visited her at Honeymoon Cottage and taken an interest in Elizabeth's writing ambitions. Mrs. Noyes's daughter had published a piece in the *Ladies Home Journal* and on her return to Washington, Mrs. Noyes had kindly sent the article on. Elizabeth was thrilled at seeing another avenue into print. Since Elizabeth had lost Mrs. Noyes's address, she asked her mother to thank her and to say how much she appreciated it—"and please don't forget!"

Surprisingly, as the wedding planning moved forward, Elizabeth received more letters than she had previously. Now that Catherine was at home more, she and her mother often put a letter each in the envelope for Elizabeth, who really appreciated them taking the time to write in the midst of the hectic activity. On one occasion, she even received a letter from her father, which, Elizabeth reported, "really overwhelmed me, and I haven't gotten over it yet."

She was so moved by his letter that she tucked it away among her treasures. In it, he addressed her as an equal, explaining his difficulties and frustrations in getting the Senate to ratify the Four Powers treaty that came out of the Washington Conference. He also wrote of his love for her and his delight in the beauty of Bermuda. Particularly, he recalled the carriage "coming around on the road to Honeymoon Cottage." That memory, he wrote, "stands out so vividly that I feel not only near you in spirit but physically—as though at any time I could sit with you by the hammock under the trees." No wonder Elizabeth told her mother that she "simply adored and was overcome" by the letter.

Mrs. Hughes also found the time to encourage Elizabeth to broaden her reading interests and had suggested she might enjoy the British author Charles Dickens. As Elizabeth lay in her hammock, she and Blanche often read aloud to each other. Now they began *Barnaby Rudge,* the first of several of Dickens's works she planned to read. The first signs were not encouraging. Elizabeth thought the only way she would "be able to stick them through is by reading exciting Western novels by Zane Grey etc with Blanche! I love western tales of ranch, lumber and cow-boy life, don't you?" Mrs. Hughes probably let this question go.

It is a testament to the depth of Elizabeth's struggle with

Dickens that she picked up Grey, as his work was not in keeping with her other reading choices. She knew all about his books, though, as they were regularly on the best-seller lists during her childhood. His novels were romantic, sometimes violent, stories of an idealized American West where good always triumphed. His accounts of the Wild West would certainly have been appealing to her even though she normally did not care for stories with lots of action.

Elizabeth persevered with Dickens out of a desire to please her mother. She resolved to "gorge my way right through" his works but would temper them with "other books that I read aloud with Blanche." Despite her stated enjoyment of Dickens's work, she did have to "make myself start" reading a new one. But start she did.

As Elizabeth's health declined, she read more and more. Fortunately, Hudson was a prolific author, and she told her mother that she had "gone on a spree" with him and was "getting loads of things read." She was not exaggerating. She also picked up books by Gene (Geneva) Stratton-Porter, another best-selling author of the early 20th century. Stratton-Porter wrote in a style similar to Hudson's and also encouraged a reverence for nature in her fiction and essays. Elizabeth read her *Homing with the Birds,* which she "just love[d]," and was eagerly looking forward to reading her novel *The Song of the Cardinal,* about the dramatic rescue of a cardinal that had been shot.

She moved from Hudson's terrain of Latin America to books about the South Pacific. She appreciated Herman Melville, who had used his own experiences at sea for his book *Typee: A Peep at Polynesian Life,* written in 1846. She also loved Joseph

Conrad's books on the South Sea Islands. Conrad had gone to sea as a young man and had originally made a name for himself as a writer of sea stories, and Elizabeth reported that she had "begun a run on him." Not surprisingly, she also snapped up two contemporary writers who published a book about their experiences in the Pacific in 1921: Charles Nordhoff and James Hall. They are known better today as the authors of *Mutiny on the Bounty,* but their first book together was *Faery Lands of the South Seas,* which they wrote after they had sailed there at the end of the war. Elizabeth was delighted by their account of "[t]hose picturesque South Sea Islanders!"

Nordhoff and Hall's book offered a few other qualities that might have added to Elizabeth's pleasure. They wrote as static observers of the world around them and they also wanted to escape confinement. For them, the confinement was of the routine of modern life and society's expectations. Both men had served as fighter pilots in World War I flying with the Escadrille Lafayette, a corps of American pilots attached to the French forces before the United States entered the war, and then with the U.S. Air Service. At war's end, they felt they had just had "the greatest adventure we shall ever know." As they sat in a café in Paris the winter of 1918, they decided that they did not want to do anything again so life-threatening but that they did crave the adventure of the "unexpected incident." So, with no ties "to drag us back to the bewilderments of modern civilization," they set sail for the South Pacific, where they found a "charmed circle" of beauty and calm. Elizabeth could identify with them for another reason. They, too, spent some of their life in the islands waiting for letters, keenly following the comings and goings of vessels, and adjusting themselves to a different pace of life.

As Elizabeth lay in her hammock, she visited others less and her world became smaller. She rested heavily on Blanche's companionship. They spent many hours together reading out loud and knitting. They had books they read together and others they read separately. Elizabeth never told her mother of Blanche's taste in reading or whether she suggested anything that Elizabeth read, though they must have discussed books. There was one popular book they had each read and enjoyed a year earlier, Louis Vance's novel *Bronze Bell*. When they were at Lake George, they went to the movies one night to see the film version and liked that too. Even though it was a romantic fiction, much of the story was set in India and had lots of detail of the country to satisfy Elizabeth's taste for news of foreign lands. Now as the two read more and more together, Blanche shared Elizabeth's journey to find her own "charmed circle" of beauty and calm.

CHARLEY BEST COULD have done with some South Sea Island tranquility. Usually he was restrained and calm, but in late March it was his turn to lose his temper. On the last day of the month, he went to Frederick Banting's rooms in a boarding house near the university to have things out with him. Work at the lab was going badly, and Best needed Banting to be fully involved again.

Banting had been a mess for a month or more. After the lab moved into high gear to produce as much of the extract as it could, his role had diminished. He fell into a funk and was so distraught that, he later recalled, "the only means by which I could get to sleep was to take alcohol." Getting it, though, was a problem. He lacked a supply and money. Prohibition had become the law in Ontario in 1918. There was a great deal of opposition to it, and the law was flaunted by those prepared to risk buying alcohol illegally. But even if he could locate some, Banting remembered, he "did not always have enough money to buy it."

He found a way around both the financial and legal impediments. The lab had plenty of alcohol on hand for experimental work. He later confessed that on a couple of occasions, he took half a liter of 95 percent proof alcohol home with him. In his rooms, he mixed it with water in the hope that he could forget his problems and sleep. He recalled that he was so distraught at the time that he did not "think there was one night during the month of March, 1922, when I went to bed sober."

It was not only feeling excluded from the action at the lab that was weighing on him; it was also his on-and-off relationship with his ex-fiancée, Edith Roach. His diary in March simply notes on one day "Edith came" and the next "Edith went." A couple of days later he received a farewell letter from her, but two days after that he called her. The young couple were torturing themselves, neither one able to break off the relationship completely. Banting went to work less and less, hiding away in his room, smoking and drinking. At least once during March, Best came to his lodgings to try and get him to leave, but to no avail.

By late on Friday evening, at the end of a long week, Best had had enough. He came again to Banting's lodgings and, this time, made a dramatic plea. The team was in crisis and needed Banting's help. Collip and the people working with him were unable to make the extract. At first, they found that when they increased the scale of the production, the substance lost its efficacy. They then went back to try to make it in extremely small quantities—but found they could not do that either. Part of the problem was that Collip had not kept meticulous notes of what he had done during his January experiments, making his method hard to replicate. A greater difficulty, though, was that in this era, the infancy of biochemistry, experiments were inherently tricky. Equipment was primitive and little was known about the substances being worked on. The slightest variation in temperature or pressure in a vacuum, for example, could lead to wildly different results. Suddenly, there was no usable extract left and no more in the pipeline. Leonard Thompson, the young diabetic receiving the extract, was sent home from Toronto General Hospital to meet his fate, as were the handful of other patients who had been receiving it. One young girl, included in this small pool because Best had got to know her family, died a few weeks later.

The group was in a panic. Apart from the terrible impact on the few recipients and the frustration they felt, they were also embarrassed. They had just published their first series of articles in Canadian academic journals describing the results on animals. There had also been a celebratory article in the *Toronto Daily Star*. The piece confidently predicted that "their discovery will be used on a large scale" in six months. Now, it seemed fortunate that this news item had merited only a small paragraph in the *New York Times* and was otherwise not widely picked up. Perhaps other papers had put it aside, jaded by the reports in earlier years of potential cures or treatments for diabetes that had come to nothing. So at least their embarrassment was confined. But the group's morale plummeted.

Now, Best stood in front of the despondent Banting and, as Banting later recalled, the young graduate student gave him a "setting out." Banting was deeply moved by Best's loyalty to him and to their work. He "thought of all the joy of the early experiments" that they had shared and agreed to pull himself together and go back to work. The two men shook hands on it. They arranged to meet at nine o'clock the next morning, "sat down and as we had done hundreds of times, planned experiments." Banting went back to "the old hard grind" and the whole group, working more as a team than they had before, set about rediscovering the secret of the extract.

In April, the four men worked hard alongside other researchers who had been brought in to help. Collip and Banting avoided each other as much as possible, but they coordinated their experiments. Anticipating that they would find the elusive substance again, Banting decided to open a private medical practice in downtown Toronto. He had not been allowed to participate in the clinical trial at Toronto General Hospital because he was not a practicing doctor, but this private practice got around that problem. In addition, he was offered an opportunity to hold a diabetes clinic at a veterans' hospital in the city. These two venues would allow him to see patients. He knew he had no experience as a clinician treating diabetics, but he was eager to see firsthand how the extract worked—and to regain some control over what he saw as his enterprise. All the scientists working on the problem were sure the extract would soon be refound, but April passed without that happening.

To add to the pressure, they had decided several weeks earlier to announce the results of their first human tests at the meeting of the Association of American Physicians in Washington, D.C., in early May. They decided to go ahead despite their present difficulty. Although all four men and their principal collaborators were listed as the paper's authors, neither Banting nor Best attended, each claiming he did not have the money to travel. None of their colleagues believed them.

At noon on May 3, 1922, John Macleod rose to speak. He laid out the group's achievements treating patients with the extract and announced for the first time a name they had only recently decided on for it: insulin. Scientists and doctors in the audience quickly realized they were listening to a paper that remade the medical landscape. Frederick Allen paid close attention and, in the discussion afterward, called it an "almost miraculous achievement." Macleod savored the acclaim and did not mention that the group no longer knew how to make it.

AS MACLEOD MADE his landmark presentation and concealed his embarrassment, Elizabeth faced her own crisis. She had weakened, and now there was an outbreak of diarrhea in the community. Unpleasant for everyone, it was a catastrophe for her. On the evening of May 3, her fever spiked at over 101 degrees and she had a bad headache. With no resistance, she was unable to recover quickly. She was ill for three weeks. For more than two of those, she was too weak to write home. When she was next able to do so, she was frank, saying, "I won't try and conceal to you what an awfully hard blow" this is. Anticipating that her mother would worry, Elizabeth chided her, "[C]heer up!! . . . I've told you the plain truth about myself, not concealing the least thing . . . there's absolutely nothing to be anxious about." Blanche, in a postscript to Elizabeth's letter, confirmed that her charge was indeed "extremely weak," but both emphasized that the crisis was over.

Neither Blanche nor Elizabeth admitted to Mrs. Hughes at the time that Elizabeth was so weak she was unable to stand up from a chair without help. They also did not reveal that she weighed less than 50 pounds.

CHAPTER 7

Born Under a Lucky Star

WITH ALL FOUR members of the Toronto research team working hard, the secret of making insulin was redis-covered in mid-May 1922. Each one contributed something toward that accomplishment, but it was Charley Best who real-ized what the final complication was: there were variations in the water pressure supplying the vacuum pumps being used, which in turn caused inconsistency in temperature and the time necessary for distillation. Finally, in a rudimentary manu-facturing system involving highly inflammatory acetone, the group managed to produce a minute quantity of insulin. Every-one heaved a sigh of relief.

There was enough now to give to a handful of diabetics. But who was to get it? In this era before universities and hospitals had ethical review boards, it was Banting himself who largely decided. Earlier, he had not been allowed to see patients when the extract was tried in the Toronto General Hospital trial because he was not a practicing doctor. But he had arranged a practice and a diabetes clinic for veterans, and he now literally had in his hands the only extract available. He could regain some control over his project. He gave a portion of the extract to Toronto General for Leonard Thompson and one or two other diabetic patients but kept the rest for those he selected.

Finding patients was not a problem. Diabetologists who had been present at the May 3 conference presentation or who kept close track of scientific research started writing to him, begging to be allowed to receive it for their patients. Because the supply was so limited and little was known about how it worked, almost all were turned away. The first injection of the rediscovered insulin went to Joe Gilchrist, Banting's friend and fellow physician, who described himself as a "human rabbit." Banting had recruited Gilchrist to work with him in the veterans' clinic and, after he reported that it worked, the two gave it to a few other very ill diabetic veterans. Otherwise, there was only enough to give to a handful of people in, or very close to, the pre-death diabetic coma, and then only if their physicians could somehow persuade Banting to give them some.

One patient in this category was 22-year-old Jim Havens, who had suffered from acute (type 1) diabetes for seven years. He was the son of James S. Havens, the vice president of the Eastman Kodak Company. When Jim was first diagnosed in 1915, his father had recently finished a term as a Democratic congressman. Mr. Havens had won a stunning electoral victory in Rochester, New York, breaking a corrupt political machine by advocating the reform platform for which then governor Charles Evans Hughes stood. In the intervening years, he had done everything possible for his son. He had taken him to

Frederick Allen and Jim had dutifully starved himself. Now, Jim was under the supervision of Dr. John Williams, a Rochester specialist, but nothing more could be done. Mr. Havens watched helplessly as his son lay near death. Jim weighed 74 pounds and wept with misery and pain.

Mr. Havens was a desperate man. He wrote of his son's plight to a friend, a Kodak store manager in Toronto, George Snowball, to find out whether there was any research being done in Canada that might help Jim. Snowball asked one of his golf partners, a fellow from the university: John Macleod. In this way, Mr. Havens heard of the promising extract and the group's problems in making it again. Dr. Williams rushed to meet Banting in Toronto. The two physicians conferred, and Banting agreed to give Williams some insulin as soon as they had a supply.

Jim Havens was the first person in the United States to get insulin, receiving his first shot on May 22, 1922. At first, he was injected with very small quantities and it had no effect. Concerned, Banting rushed to Rochester. Jim later remembered that Banting arrived with "insulin in his pocket" and discovered they just needed to use more. The next day Jim was sugar free, more cheerful, without pain, and able to sit in a chair reading. Over the next few weeks, his insulin was sent on the five P.M. train from Toronto in the hands of a kindly porter. Jim still ate only about 900 calories a day, experienced terrible sores around the injection site due to the insulin's impurities, and stayed weak, but he was in much better spirits. His transformation was so great that Dr. Williams wrote that he found it "difficult to record in temperate language."

Mr. and Mrs. Havens were thrilled that Banting had saved their son and, during his brief visit to their home, they quickly arranged a dinner for him to meet George Eastman, the wealthy founder of the Kodak Company. Eastman wanted to recruit Banting to work at the new medical school at the University of Rochester, but Banting preferred to stay in Canada and declined.

Eastman had every reason to hope Banting could be tempted. Since the conference presentation and the rediscovery, Banting's professional star was rising and he was open about being frustrated with the resources available to him in Toronto. Eastman's offer was one of several that he seriously considered. The University of Toronto had to respond quickly with an offer of their own to keep Banting and insulin in the city. They did. By late June, Banting had secured a well-paid appointment in the university's Department of Medicine and a diabetic clinic that would start at Toronto General Hospital in the fall.

In the meantime, it was imperative to solve the problem of insulin production. Not only were diabetics in desperate need, but also a meaningful body of clinical evidence could hardly be gathered with such a small pool of recipients. Jim Havens's experience showed that the researchers did not know how much to use or what the patient's new diet should be. The knowledge that giving too much could be fatal also made them cautious. Diabetologists such as Elliott Joslin, Frederick Allen, and the New Yorker H. Rawle Geyelin had lots of what Geyelin called "clinical material" they could supervise in trials. They were also highly skilled clinicians and had much more experience than Banting in monitoring and measuring patients' responses.

The data they could collect would answer many of the questions about how insulin should be used but, without a steady, reliable supply, they could not begin to gather it.

The Toronto group and the university's Connaught Laboratories realized that they did not have the resources to solve the problem and, finally, George Clowes's perseverance paid off. The Canadians handed the problem to Eli Lilly & Company to solve. In return, when it succeeded, Lilly would have a one-year monopoly on insulin manufacture in the United States and Central and South America and then would make it under license under the same terms and conditions that governed other manufacturers. The agreement required that the team patent insulin. Banting and Macleod, as medical men, were concerned about the ethics of doing that, so it was agreed that Collip and Best would apply for the patent, then when it was granted, immediately transfer it to the university, which they did. At the beginning of June, Best and Collip headed to Indianapolis, where the company was based, to teach the Lilly chemists all they knew about making insulin. Everyone hoped that Lilly would soon find the key to the production problem.

With that task handed over and the academic year at an end, the group broke up. Best came back to Toronto and then at the end of June left for a long vacation with his family in Maine. Collip, his Rockefeller fellowship over, returned with his family to Calgary and the University of Alberta, to become chair of the Department of Biochemistry. Macleod, too, left town. He headed out to a facility in New Brunswick to do research there on the potential for using fish as a source of insulin.

With his colleagues gone, Banting was frantically busy. Insulin production continued at a snail's pace in Toronto, and he juggled the scant supply among a few diabetics. He met with diabetologists, trying to learn as much as possible about treating patients, not something he knew very much about, and still flirted with other job opportunities. And he decided who could and could not get insulin.

ELIZABETH WAS NOT at death's door—yet. Despite her attack of diarrhea at the beginning of May, her ability to tolerate food without sugar spilling into her urine was improving slightly and she was able to eat a little more. Her diet now included an occasional grapefruit, strawberry, and piece of fish ("needless to say not at the same meal"). And now on her half days, she added milk to her cocoa and had a vegetable with her single piece of meat and was "mighty glad." But she was weaker, and spent more and more hours in the hammock.

One day in mid-May, she opened a letter from her mother and read some interesting news. Mrs. Hughes had seen a newspaper item about the great breakthrough in diabetic research at the University of Toronto. She cut it out and sent it to Elizabeth. Elizabeth was excited to see it and was able to send some other news back about it from another source. Blanche was friendly with another Joslin-trained nurse working in Bermuda, Miss Mckay, who cared for an older American woman who had "mild" (type II) diabetes. Elizabeth did not see very much of the patient, but Miss Mckay regularly came to visit on her days off and Elizabeth liked her. Miss Mckay had heard about the discovery from Joslin himself. Elizabeth told her mother that the eminent physician thought it "the greatest step that has ever been taken so far." "Isn't that perfectly wonderful?" she wrote. "And you know when he praises something it's sure to be worthwhile for he's exceptionally particular." Blanche added a postscript to Elizabeth's letter home, commenting on the news. She agreed that it seemed that doctors were "at last really finding a cure for diabetes" but tempered her optimism. She hoped it would, at least, allow patients to live on "a more normal diet and gain in strength."

There was no more news about the discovery in the days that followed. Guided by Blanche, Elizabeth restrained her more excited thoughts. Perhaps it just seemed too remote. She did not dwell on what insulin might mean to her and never referred to it again in the weeks that followed.

Mrs. Hughes, meanwhile, received mixed signals from Elizabeth about her condition. The diarrhea had been a significant setback for her. Blanche was so worried that she had written to Dr. Allen, who now wanted to see his patient to do some blood tests when they returned to the United States. But Elizabeth's letters were upbeat, rushing past news of her frailty and instead dwelling on the new foods she was eating, her improved tolerances, her reading, and other activities. Elizabeth had even suggested that her parents meet her in New York when she sailed back so they could "spree" in the city for a few days.

One of the reasons for Elizabeth's cheery tone was that she knew her mother was under enormous pressure in the month of June. Catherine's wedding was on June 10. There were only 100 or so guests at the service in the Bethlehem Chapel of Washington National Cathedral, but many more were invited to the reception at the Pan American Union building, which was decorated now not only with flags but with "pink roses and larkspur." Catherine was, the *New York Times* noted, "the first cabinet bride of this administration," and the event "one of the most notably interesting weddings of many seasons." The plans for it filled the society pages in the New York and Washington papers for weeks. To add to the pressure, there was no respite from official duties. Catherine and her parents attended a White House garden party for veterans just two days before the wedding.

The big day dawned. The ceremony was, of course, a family affair. Secretary Hughes gave away his daughter. Catherine looked lovely in a crepe-backed satin gown of "long loose lines so much in vogue just now," according to the Washington *Evening Star,* with a bodice embroidered with pearls. Her brother Charles's two little boys were her train bearers, her sister-in-law, Marjorie, was a maid of honor, and brother Charles was an usher. Mrs. Hughes, in a beige georgette and lace dress with a lavender sash and matching hat, kept a watchful eye on the proceedings, enjoying the calm before the reception to follow. Once there, she and Mr. Hughes and the bride and groom welcomed "several thousand" guests to celebrate the event. The president and Mrs. Harding were the most important of these, and they held up the receiving line for more than ten minutes while they chatted with the newlyweds. Everyone recognized this compliment to the happy couple even though it meant they could not greet their other guests for a while.

Elizabeth and Blanche sent a congratulatory telegram to Catherine and Chauncey. Otherwise, they contented themselves with reading the details of the event from Mrs. Hughes and the newspaper reports. Elizabeth must have been a little bit jealous that even her little nephews had participated. And she would have liked to share the family's annoyance that, even though the *Post* reported the wedding prominently on page two, it spelled Catherine's name with a "K" in the headline.

But this was not the only tumultuous event for the Hugheses in June. The Vassar classmates of their deceased daughter, Helen, had built a memorial chapel to honor her at Silver Bay on Lake George, where she had done some of her Y.W.C.A. work and near where she had died. That memorial was unveiled on June 25, just two weeks after the wedding.

Knowing about these stressful events, it was hardly surprising that Elizabeth kept the focus of her letters away from any bad news about herself. She told her parents she would "be thinking of you" at Helen's memorial and although "not there in body" would be there "with all my heart and soul." She quickly reverted to her usual cheery tone and encouraged her mother not to get too worn out with it all.

Mrs. Hughes took Elizabeth's reports of her health at face value. Having myriad demands on her time and wallet, she sat down just after Catherine's wedding and curtailed Elizabeth's plans. On the grounds of cost alone, she dismissed the idea of lingering in New York and thought the trip to Dr. Allen's unnecessary given that Elizabeth had recovered from her setback and her diet seemed to be going well. She instructed Elizabeth and Blanche to return directly to Washington.

Elizabeth was chastened. She agreed that, since, "as you say, I am getting on so nicely," she did not need to go to the doctor:

Dr. Allen's fees are perfectly dreadful of course, and it just hurts me when I think of them, and the awful amount of money you are paying out for me all the time. You don't realize how much I appreciate all that and how I want, if I can, in my small way help to reduce it. So I hate to think of having to go out there and I don't want you to think I do and also to think that I'm not thankful and appreciative of all you're doing for me, for I certainly am, and can never in my life feel grateful enough for being born with such marvelous parents! How can I ever repay you? I never can, I'm afraid, but I want you to know that if I ever could, I would with all my heart and soul and voice!

But she was soon to arrive home, and she did not want her parents to be shocked when they saw her. She tried to strike a balance between being reassuring and truthful. "My diet's going beautifully," she began, "but as yet I am still terrible about climbing stairs and getting out of chairs etc." But she was exercising, "and as far as plain walking and doing things is concerned my strength is absolutely returned." Still, she was concerned that her mother would be shocked at her weakness. "[Y]ou mustn't be surprised at it, that's all, when I see you." This probably left Antoinette no wiser.

HAD MRS. HUGHES not been distracted by June's tumultuous social events, she might have picked up on one clue to Elizabeth's real condition: her activities, or rather her lack of them. These changed dramatically in the weeks following her illness. She went from going out and about in the carriage sightseeing and visiting to spending hours in the garden hammock. Mrs. Hughes may have thought that Elizabeth was simply heeding her advice to rest more. But in fact, Elizabeth was now too frail to get out much. It was no longer from a beach or scenic point that she wrote about enjoying the scenery or a sunset. Rather, it was from the hammock that she described the balmy weather, the brightly colored cardinals flying around, which she thought were "the cutest things," and the blossoming oleander.

It was from the confines of her garden that she celebrated the flowers of the islands. She told her mother, "I'm getting to love flowers now just as much as my passion for birds & trees etc. & Oh, how I love this place so full of them. . . . Everyday new flowers burst out now—new trees are blossoming . . . and I'm just living in a thrill of ecstasy all the time." Every day, she wrote, "grows more heavenly."

Like other visitors, she was especially struck by the oleander. She had probably never seen the plant before coming to Bermuda, as it needs a temperate climate and had only been introduced in the United States to places such as Florida and South Carolina. Native to the Mediterranean and southwest Asia, it had been brought to the islands in the late 18th century and thrived, as it can cope easily with sandy soil and salty air.

Elizabeth could not help but notice it. Growing up to 30 feet in height, the plants have thick clusters of flowers in red, pink, yellow, or white, and were used as windbreaks around many homes and gardens. Despite its beauty, every part of the oleander is very poisonous and it has to be handled carefully, but it is stunning to look at. In early 1922, the *Royal Gazette* reported that some oleanders on the island were struck by a mysterious blight and the government had begun spraying to counter it. However, near Elizabeth's cottage there was no problem, and the plants were "unbelievably beautiful—just weighed down and overladen with blossoms."

Elizabeth also enjoyed many other flowers. By the end of the 19th century lilies and lily bulbs had become an important island export, and everywhere she turned there were "fields and fields of beautiful blooming Easter lilies." She and Blanche were thrilled when some American friends leaving the island invited them to help themselves to flowers from their garden. They were able to pick "roses, sweet peas, nasturtians [*sic*] and lilies and now we're just a bower of flowers in every room, besides being very sweet too." Elizabeth loved them so much that she wanted to press the petals in a book to preserve them, but they turned moldy. Blanche had the idea of preserving them in candle wax, which Elizabeth found "lots of fun to do."

Resting in her hammock or bedroom, her enjoyment of the natural world intensified. Her letters became filled with details not of what she was going out to see but what was coming to the garden. Always an eager bird watcher, she was particularly enchanted by the bright red cardinals, which came very close to her window. She heard cardinals and bluebirds "calling their various mating notes." Optimistically, she "hung some calabashes," gourds, with seeds near the door to draw them near the cottage. Her effort paid off. One morning,

a pair of cardinals came right near my window, saw it and immediately sat one on each side eating the seed and chirping that "chirp" as they did so. Oh I nearly died as you can well imagine, for they were so beautiful, cute & tame. Isn't it just too lovely that they'll do that and so near the house too? I was overcome with delight, for you know how I adore them!

She continued to take great pleasure in art and music — delights that required little energy to enjoy. She could not hear her beloved Mme. Homer, of course; the famous contralto was still in New York. But Elizabeth enjoyed listening to an occasional military band concert in the park. The *Royal Gazette* reported that these performances by the East Lancashire Regimental band struck "the most distinctive note in our social life, being appreciated alike by visitors and residents." At one of these concerts, Elizabeth was especially pleased when the band played "the dear little 'Birthday Serenade' that Helen loved so, so beautifully." The piece, by American composer Katharine Lucke, brought back many memories of her sister.

Unable to go out much, she surrounded herself with photographs of the Bermudian scenery. She had tried to record it herself, taking small black-and-white images with her little box camera, but it was too basic to take very satisfying photographs of the vistas she had seen. She preferred to have larger, professional color images of the landscape. She used some of her Christmas money from her mother to buy two colored photographs (made using the recently developed autochrome technique) by a local artist, Stuart Hayward. To her great delight, when the Bermuda Trade Development Board was courting her after her father's visit, they gave her eight more Hayward prints. She felt she had been "born under a lucky star" to receive such bounty. The only shadow was that the board was going to print her letter of thanks in their newsletter. ("Horrors!") But she told her mother not to worry. She would write a "careful" note and "try not to disgrace you." The Hayward prints now went above the fireplace so she could look at them every day.

This pleasure in beauty even extended to everyday items such as clothing and knickknacks. She enjoyed the look of her collection of "dangles, beads etc." She loved the touch of a dress she had made of pongee silk and of "wonderful white deerskin gauntlet gloves" that she bought. She admired the look and feel of a "Roman sash" that Catherine had brought her back from Europe.

As she became increasingly immobilized, this intense delight brought her a great deal of solace. People suffering from chronic illness and many others suffering from a variety of soul-destroying experiences have found beauty to be a life preserver. Viktor Frankl, the psychiatrist and former inmate of Auschwitz, cited beauty in all its forms as an important source of comfort to him and others. He broke down the elements that provided comfort into two kinds: those that generated what he called "negative happiness," or happiness rooted in being free from pain or suffering, and those that were "real, positive pleasures." One of these positive pleasures, he observed, came from an "intensification of inner life" in which people "experienced the beauty of art and nature as never before."

It was this intensification that now sustained Elizabeth. She never ceased to suffer, though she may have become accustomed to her trials, but she took a positive pleasure in beauty in its many forms, sights, sounds, and textures.

WEAK AS SHE WAS, Elizabeth did not completely withdraw from the world. She continued to meet friends old and new. Colonel Swalm, the congenial American consul, took Elizabeth and Blanche with him to visit a U.S. Navy cruiser that had arrived in Hamilton. They were greeted by a visiting admiral as well as the ship's captain. However, being 14 years old, the highlight of Elizabeth's day was getting a tour of the ship from "an awfully nice, handsome midshipman." It was, she wrote, an "absolute red-letter day."

She had a great time also when she had the chance to entertain an old friend from New York. One day, the phone rang and it was her pal Connie McLane, the 14-year-old daughter of New York businessman and civic leader Thomas McLane and his wife, Mary. Elizabeth was delighted to discover that the family was in Bermuda for a week. The two girls knew each other from the Brearley School in New York and had not seen each other since Elizabeth moved to Washington the previous year. Connie came over for lunch and the afternoon, and Elizabeth quickly discovered "she's just the same sweet old Connie McLane she always was." The two chatted for hours, and Connie also joined Elizabeth on a sightseeing tour another day. The two had lots to catch up on: "if we didn't make our tongues go, nobody could!" It was a lovely visit.

She longed for more company from friends her age such as Connie, but not all girls could accept her circumstances. Claudia and Dorothy Duran were twins she had met through

Guides and at first she had greatly enjoyed their company. But one day, when they came to visit "they were very rude and unmannerly at the table about my food." The final straw for Elizabeth was when Blanche observed them in Hamilton "standing on the streets downtown talking to young men." It was one thing for Elizabeth to enjoy the company of a sailor to whom she had been introduced; it was another for the Duran twins to chat with men they did not know in public. Elizabeth described them as "fly-away, light girls" and was so disgusted that she told her mother she was "not going to continue to keep up with them from now on."

Fortunately, other Guide friends still enriched her life. In June, she took Gwen Simmons, the daughter of a British officer on the island and a "sincere, lovable" girl, and two Guide leaders out for a moonlight sail. Gwen later spent the night, as they were not back until after ten o'clock, and she stayed to chat the next morning. Elizabeth was thrilled.

Sailing was a new activity for her, and that she pursued it in her weakened state is a testament both to her love of the sport and her desire, weak as she was, for some adventure. A family friend had arranged her first sail in April and when Elizabeth wrote to her mother about it, the news required a great many exclamation marks. She had gone out of her cottage to find the boat "waiting at the dock to take us out sailing!!! Imagine it!!! My first sail, and if I didn't have more fun than I can put into words!" The weather had been windy and the sea rough. Her face, hands, and hair were soaked by spray. She loved it. "Oh boy," she wrote, "was there ever anything like it, and it was so much more fun it being rough and sporty!"

She could not wait to go again and so made an important decision. Elizabeth had enough in her budget to hire a carriage and driver for an excursion once a week. Now, she decided to hire a boat and captain and "take my 'weekly drive' so to speak in sailing instead." Unfortunately, due to her diarrhea, she was too weak to go for several weeks, but in late May she went out again and "the water was just rough enough to get us plenty wet and give us numerous rolls and slides, and oh I simply reveled in it."

That she was able to enjoy sailing in these conditions while so weak is astonishing. She was so frail that she would not have been able to brace herself as the boat heeled on the water. She would have needed to be tied in and have someone holding her. That did not deter her; she had always been eager for spills and thrills. At Lake George she had loved going out on the *Snark,* a friend's motorboat, even though she wished "it went a bit faster." That same summer, she had also begged her parents to allow her to go up joyriding in an airplane. Lake George, like other resort areas, had regular summer visits from aerialists or barnstormers. These traveling air shows were a way that many pilots, male and female, made a living in the 1920s. "[O]h couldn't you please let me go up!" Elizabeth had begged in a letter. But her parents refused. She would have loved to do an "aerial tour" in Bermuda, too, but knew better than to ask a second time.

From the hammock, she made plans for her future travels. "I'm so happy when I think of coming here again next year," she told her mother. So she did not feel sad at leaving Honeymoon Cottage at the end of June, knowing she would soon be back. And she knew that she would be up in Lake George again in late August; that visit had just been planned. Elizabeth and Blanche were to go there when Mrs. Hughes accompanied her husband to Brazil to join the celebrations of the centennial of that country's independence. Elizabeth, who of course longed to travel, could hardly contain herself when she heard about her mother's proposed Latin American adventure. It made her "an absolute wreck!" with excitement. How she wished that her mother could "tuck Blanche & I away on that destroyer" they were sailing on! She could not go, of course, and knew it. She dutifully accepted the visit to Lake George as her consolation prize. The lake, she wrote to her mother, "always means heaven to me," and she and Blanche would have a wonderful time there.

As the stay in Bermuda wound down, Elizabeth gamely picked up another work by Charles Dickens, this time *Bleak House*. And she began it on her half day, when she was eating only 350 calories—a bold move. She was always surprised, she wrote, at how good his books were, "but my, what a bore to start."

Blanche packed their trunks for the sail home. Elizabeth wanted to say good-bye to the two men who had made her stay in Bermuda so enjoyable, Governor Willcocks and Colonel Swalm. Governor Willcocks and his wife were also leaving. His term as governor was over and they were returning to England as Elizabeth herself departed, so Elizabeth would not see them when she returned the following winter. She could not say good-bye to Colonel Swalm in person. The aged consul had fallen ill and was taken to the hospital in mid-June. Elizabeth sent flowers and worried about him but was unable to visit.

She knew that when she visited Bermuda again, it would be a very different place without their company.

AS ELIZABETH MADE preparations for her journey home, Banting was bombarded by requests from doctors seeking insulin for desperately ill patients, but it was still in critically short supply. Lilly chemists worked hard trying to increase the scale of production but so far had had no success. They still found that the extract lost its efficacy when it was made in larger quantities.

To complicate matters, the small amount of insulin being made in Toronto was of very poor quality, as Jim Havens now discovered to his cost. Since receiving it, he had been able to sit in his room in the family home on East Avenue in Rochester, chat with his older sister and younger siblings, and enjoy life once again. But his progress was halting. The sores around the injection site were sometimes so bad that Dr. Williams had to withhold insulin for a couple of days to allow Jim to recover.

In July, the quality of the Toronto insulin became so poor it almost killed him. Williams wrote to Banting, "I thought he would die on me. He appeared to be heading for coma." The patient had "a sensation all over his body as though he had been poisoned." Fortunately, Jim survived this, but he remained very weak and dropped back to his pre-insulin weight. Fortunately, Clowes and the Lilly chemists had a small, better-quality amount they could give to Banting, and Jim did not have a second such experience.

Despite the inconsistent quality of the insulin and a supply so limited they were taking it away from one person to give to

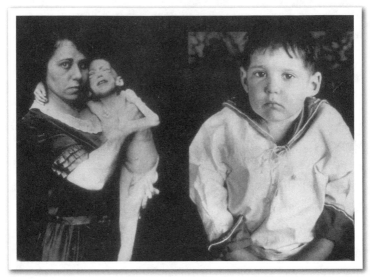

*The shocking before and after-insulin photographs of a three-year-old,
15-pound diabetic child identified only as J.L. Courtesy Eli Lilly and
Company Archives.*

another, Banting added a few more patients to the roster. He
agreed to give it to a woman who was a patient of a Toronto
doctor, L. C. Palmer. Palmer had a special claim to Banting's
goodwill. He had been a fellow medical officer alongside Banting during the war, and the two had been together at the front
line just before the Battle of Cambrai in which Banting had
won his Military Cross. Palmer's request for insulin for a needy
patient was not one that Banting could ignore.

He also gave in to a request for an eight-year-old American
girl, Ruth Whitehill, who was brought to Toronto by her mother
from Baltimore, near death. And he gave permission for Mildred
Ryder to bring her six-year-old son, Teddy, with her from New
Jersey. He weighed only 25 pounds. His uncle, Morton Ryder, a

doctor, had gone to Toronto in the spring to meet Banting hoping to get access to insulin, without success. But Banting held out hope for some later. At the end of June, Dr. Ryder wrote a pleading letter to Banting. "We must not delay," he argued, "if the boy's life is to be saved." Banting relented.

MEANWHILE, ELIZABETH MADE her way home from Bermuda. When the steamship *Fort Hamilton* docked in New York, she was exhausted from her journey. Despite that, she was determined to leave the ship unaided and walk down the gangway under her own steam. She did it. For someone who could do little more than "ordinary walking" on her best day, this was a real accomplishment.

On July 1, she and Blanche traveled on to Union Station in Washington, where they were met by her parents. Mr. and Mrs. Hughes, worn out from Catherine's wedding, the unveiling of Helen's memorial, and a great many public commitments, were looking forward to seeing Elizabeth. In the light of her generally upbeat tone from Bermuda, the good news about her diet, and the encouraging breakthrough in diabetic research, they probably anticipated her return with hearts that were somewhat light.

The reality of seeing her must have been shocking.

Antoinette Hughes now joined the families petitioning Banting. She knew that the discovery had taken place at the University of Toronto and had seen Banting's name in the paper. She went straight to the source. She wrote to him on July 3, 1922. Elizabeth had, she wrote, "despite our care, gotten into this exceedingly weak and wasted condition." Her daughter was "pitifully depleted and reduced. She is five feet tall and weighs less than fifty pounds." She did not identify herself as the wife of the American secretary of state but made the connection clear when she asked that Banting reply to her care of the State Department. She petitioned on Elizabeth's behalf, she wrote, for two reasons. The first was Elizabeth's terrible physical state. The other was her virtue. "She is a model patient," her mother argued, "having never once in these three years gone over her diet. The steps backward—when they have come—have invariably been due to no fault of hers and we feel that this strength of character—which her nurse considers quite unusual—is—of course—much in her favor." Mrs. Hughes hoped that Banting could help them. But he could not. There was very little insulin available and he could not predict when more would be.

Mrs. Hughes was heartsick at the news and asked Banting to keep the family in mind "should you have any particularly good news" about a future supply. As a physician friend of Macleod's observed as he unsuccessfully pleaded with him on behalf of a diabetic patient, it was hard for insulin to "be in sight, yet not in reach."

But as her parents despaired, Elizabeth made plans for her writing career. Shortly before she left Bermuda, she had commissioned a local cabinetmaker to make a small cedar writing desk that she could balance on her lap. It was 20 inches by 12, "just a nice size to write on, on my lap and to hold things . . . and not a bit heavy." It was perfect for when she felt too tired to sit at a table.

There was another purchase she needed to make that was essential to a budding author. She hoped to use her savings, all 25 dollars, to buy "one of those small traveling typewriters." Before she left Bermuda, she pleaded for permission with all the expertise a 14-year-old can bring to bear: "I'm simply dying for one! It would mean so much to me now in writing all my manuscripts and letters etc besides being lots of fun to work. Anyway authors always have one, and though I'm beginning early, I nevertheless want one, and I'd learn to manage it correctly!" Elizabeth bought the typewriter promptly after her return.

She quickly settled into Greystone, the house at Rock Creek, which her parents had rented again for the summer. In early July, the women of the household were all busy. Blanche unpacked. Mrs. Hughes wrote her desperate plea to Banting. And Elizabeth noted in her diet records that she now weighed "48 ¼ dressed."

CHAPTER 8

The Shot Heard Round
the World

I N JULY 1922, Elizabeth lay in Greystone, the Hugheses' summer home in Rock Creek Park. Every aspect of her appearance reflected her depleted and malnourished condition. Her
skin was dry and cracked and her hair was limp. She had little
energy. Even "plain walking" was now difficult for her. Everyone
around her knew that she was slipping away.

Her father continued to immerse himself in work. He was
absorbed with diplomatic initiatives for reducing tensions with
Cuba, Brazil, Mexico, and other Latin American nations, to
repair some of the damage done to relations by various American interventions in the region. He hosted a Chilean–Peruvian
conference to ease tensions between those two countries, and
prepared for his trip to Brazil in late August to join the celebrations for the centennial of its independence.

Mrs. Hughes stayed home more than usual. The formal

social season had ended for the summer and many of the Washington elite had left town. But there were still a number of events to occupy her time and mind. She and her husband attended a large dinner the French ambassador threw to celebrate Bastille Day, commemorating the French Revolution. A week later, the Hugheses hosted yet another large reception at the Pan American Union building. This one marked the end of the Chilean–Peruvian conference and was another "brilliant" event according to the *Post*. She also stayed busy planning future events, particularly those of the women's auxiliary of the Pan American Scientific Congress, scheduled to meet in Washington in October. But apart from these demands on her time, she spent many anxious hours around Elizabeth.

The Hugheses were at a difficult juncture in coping with their sick child. They could see her dramatic deterioration, but she had already lived with diabetes longer than anyone had predicted and might go on to live for months more. Should they bring their lives to a halt just in case this was the end? Or carry on normally, continuing their work and social obligations? Doing the latter would provide stability and structure for themselves and Elizabeth as they watched and waited to see whether she failed further over the summer.

But they could not drift along indefinitely. In this era before easy air travel, their planned trip to Brazil would require a lengthy sea voyage and an absence of a month. The Hugheses would be in touch with the State Department using what the *New York Times* called "war radio service." This connected ships to radio relay stations along the coast of the United States and West Indies. So Mr. and Mrs. Hughes would hear news of Elizabeth but they could not quickly return in the event of an emergency.

Should Mrs. Hughes accompany her husband? She hesitated. Two months earlier, Mr. Hughes had committed to the trip and she had anticipated joining him. Privately, they made plans for Elizabeth to go to Lake George in their absence, but there had been no public announcement of Mrs. Hughes's intentions. Now they did not know whether Mrs. Hughes should leave, or even if Elizabeth was strong enough to travel again.

Finally, the Hugheses took their cue from Elizabeth. Weak and wasted as she was, she became no worse in July. They made their decision. In early August, the State Department announced that Mrs. Hughes would "definitely" accompany her husband to Brazil in late August.

AS JULY CAME to an end, Frederick Banting, the lone member of the team to stay in Toronto that summer, continued his hectic whirl. He treated the few patients for whom he had insulin, fought for better equipment for his Toronto lab, raised funds elsewhere when the university was not forthcoming, and resisted the lure of money from the various job offers that came his way. He found time in his busy schedule to spend hours with his private patients, eight-year-old Ruth Whitehill and six-year-old Teddy Ryder. Even though he wrote about them in his medical notes in a detached, clinical way, his interactions with them and their families were warm. He was happy to chat and be drawn out about his own worries.

He also traveled to Indianapolis to visit the Lilly chemists and discovered that they had greatly improved on the Toronto group's makeshift manufacturing techniques. Some of these changes came from having more people, resources, and sophisticated equipment; others came from innovations in the production process such as switching to pork pancreas from beef and removing the alcohol used in preparing the solution by a vacuum distillation technique. The quality of Lilly's insulin was a bit more consistent, and Toronto now began to copy the Indianapolis manufacturing methods. In early August, George Clowes, Lilly's research director, and his staff were able to make insulin in slightly larger quantities. Clinical trials could begin.

Because there was so much about the drug that was unknown, Clowes and Banting decided to restrict the trials to the patients of a small group of diabetologists who could study in detail its impact under variable circumstances. Banting, a few physicians at Toronto General Hospital, and a hand-picked group of other diabetic specialists including Frederick Allen, Elliott Joslin, Rawle Geyelin, and John Williams, would get enough for some of their patients. They had to be conservative about to whom they gave it. Supplies were still tight but slowly increasing. By the end of the year, several hundred diabetics would be able to receive it.

Events moved quickly. On August 6, 1922, Joslin entered his clinic to give the first shot to one of his patients. He had been so excited at the prospect that the night before he was unable to sleep. The recipient was a 42-year-old woman who weighed 69 pounds, "just about the weight of her bones and a human soul," he later recalled.

Frederick Allen was not long behind him. Allen arrived in Toronto on August 8 to advise Banting on diet for insulin recipients and to collect his own supply. He returned to his clinic in Morristown, New Jersey, on August 10. There, one of Allen's nurses, Margate Kienast, remembered that a few of his sickest patients, frail and anxious, awaited his return. They felt "intolerable hope" as they listened for the sound of his footsteps in the hallway. When Allen entered, he appeared profoundly moved by the desperate faces that greeted him and simply said to them, "I think I have something for you."

Elizabeth was not among Allen's patients that day. She surely would have been had the family wanted it. But the Hugheses preferred that Elizabeth go to Toronto—"the fountainhead," as she later called it—to receive insulin. Allen and perhaps others had lobbied Banting to attend to Elizabeth personally. There was an exchange of telegrams between Banting and the Hugheses and by August 12, it had been decided. Elizabeth would travel to Canada.

It is not clear whether the Hugheses knew of the availability of insulin when they decided that Mrs. Hughes would go to Brazil. Her decision to travel was made by August 5, at approximately the time Joslin and Allen knew they would imminently have the drug. Still, with Elizabeth's condition weak but stable and insulin a highly experimental treatment, it is unlikely the news of its availability swayed their decision.

But several days passed between their discovering that insulin was available and their decision to send Elizabeth to Toronto. Perhaps they hesitated because the journey itself was a gamble. It might be too much for her. She would have to travel by train to New York, a trip of several hours, and there change for the 12-hour journey to Toronto, and all this as a summer

heat wave gripped the Northeast. Perhaps they needed to convince Banting to treat her. There were other doctors with desperate patients begging him for the drug; he did not need to
include a girl from a prominent American family who could get
it from Allen. But the Hugheses and Banting were able to reach
an agreement. Elizabeth would be treated in Toronto.

Allen was delighted to hear the news. He wrote to Banting
as soon as Mr. Hughes telegraphed him. "You will," Allen told
Banting, "find Elizabeth a model patient in all respects." Not
only was her nurse, Blanche Burgess, "especially qualified in
this work, but also Elizabeth herself has a thorough knowledge
of all details of the diet." Elizabeth, Allen wrote, deserved Banting's care in her own right, "in addition to any consideration
due on account of her family."

Mrs. Hughes had not a moment to spare. She had just
enough time to take Elizabeth and Blanche to Canada and
return home before leaving for South America. On August 14,
the three boarded the train at Washington's Union Station, and
they arrived in Toronto the next day. Antoinette took Elizabeth
to meet Banting right away.

In his notes, he described the skeletal child before him.
She was, he wrote, slightly under five feet tall and weighed
45 pounds, "extremely emaciated . . . skin dry & scaly, hair brit-
tle & thin, abdomen prommt [prominent], shoulders drooped,
muscles extremely wasted, subcutaneous tissues almost completely absorbed. She was scarcely able to walk on account of
weakness." In short, her condition was shocking. Elizabeth
received her first shot of insulin the next day, August 16, three
days before her 15th birthday.

Mrs. Hughes could not linger to see the results. She installed Elizabeth and Blanche in a small apartment at 78 Grosvenor Street, a short walk from the university, and arrived back in Washington a couple of days later. She and Mr. Hughes were leaving on August 23 for New York and setting sail for Brazil the following day. A formal departure photograph taken for the *Washington Post* at Union Station shows Mrs. Hughes looking elegant as ever. Only those who knew her well would have noticed how tired she looked, not surprising given that she had just traveled more than 1,200 miles in a week and set her daughter off on an unknown journey.

Mrs. Hughes knew the debt she owed Banting for making it possible for her to continue with her plans. As she packed her trunk, she received a letter from him updating her on Elizabeth's progress. Mrs. Hughes quickly wrote back, telling him that the good news he related "gives me confidence to leave her in your care and to feel that she and Mrs. Burgess are so comfortably settled." On behalf of herself and her husband, she expressed her gratitude and "deep appreciation" for all he was doing. The Hugheses set sail knowing Elizabeth was in safe hands.

THE FIRST FEW DAYS Elizabeth was on insulin, Banting had her follow the kind of conservative diet that Allen, Joslin, and other clinicians had recommended. They advocated using insulin carefully, letting the patient adjust, increasing food intake slowly, and monitoring every morsel ingested to see how the body responded. No one knew how much diabetics could or should eat. Diabetologists erred on the side of caution, giving insulin in small amounts and calibrating the diet to match it.

Elizabeth lived this way for her first ten days on insulin. She ate between 1,100 and 1,200 calories a day, more than she had eaten since her diagnosis, without any half or fast days. She was delighted, especially at being able to enjoy a larger variety of vegetables and fruits, eating plentiful amounts of such things as tomatoes, peaches, eggplant, and cauliflower. On her wasted frame, this caloric intake was enough for her to put on seven pounds in the same period.

But Banting developed a bold idea. He soon had a bit more insulin available and he decided to throw caution to the wind. His colleagues were constrained by their years of experience as clinicians, keeping diabetics alive with starvation therapy. Banting, in contrast, had barely seen a diabetic until a few months before. Now, with Elizabeth, a starving, emaciated child, standing before him and enough insulin in his possession, he decided simply to feed her. He would give her enough insulin to match the food she consumed. He knew he was doing something unconventional, so he asked Elizabeth to be discreet. Elizabeth told her mother before she boarded the ship for Brazil that the new diet was "our great big secret!" Allen would "have ten fits if he knew." Even though the secret diet had not begun yet, she was optimistic and thought it might allow her to "lead a normal existence with Blanche to take care of my diet."

On August 25, Elizabeth started eating just over 2,000 calories a day. She told her mother she would be drinking "about a pint of heavy cream a day if I can find room for it." She found room. Things went so well that after a few days, Banting increased her food intake to about 2,500 calories. She breakfasted one day on "two peaches, almost a whole shredded wheat with 4 ounces of heavy cream, an egg, bacon, cream cheese, lots of butter, and best of all a whole slice of bread toasted, on which I spread my butter and cheese." Allen would indeed have had ten fits if he had known.

So would the other specialists giving insulin to their patients. While Elizabeth was tucking into this feast, Jim Havens in Rochester, for example, still ate a very restricted diet. Only after he had been on insulin for more than six months was he allowed to enjoy his first egg on toast in years. It was such a highlight, he wrote to Banting about it jokingly as "an historical event." Jim was thrilled because the simple dish was "my idea of the only food necessary in heaven." His father and doctor were equally excited. "Dad and Dr. Williams grouped around me in a half circle and watched."

Toast, slathered in butter, was already old news to Elizabeth. She regularly ate that, liver, veal, chicken, salmon, orange juice, melons, grapes, potatoes—and more cream. "I could use up pages," she told her mother excitedly, "just innumerating [sic] all the dishes I have nowadays, and it seems to me that I eat something everyday that I haven't tasted for over three years, and you don't know how good it seems and how much I appreciate every morsel I eat."

Despite this joy that she surely felt, it is likely that, after her starvation therapy, Elizabeth found it physically hard to consume this quantity of food, yet she never complained. After four short weeks on this diet, she weighed about 65 pounds, an increase of almost 45 percent since she had arrived in Toronto.

NOT SURPRISINGLY, her body responded right away to this nourishment. Even she could see the dramatic physical changes. "I simply don't recognize myself as the same person when I look in the mirror," she wrote. "Its [*sic*] simply killing too when I go out anywhere and see people I haven't seen for a week say, they simply stare at me in perfect wonder." One acquaintance, a Mrs. Chambers, "kept staring at me fixedly until she burst out with 'Gracious how that girl has changed.' ... Its [*sic*] like that everywhere I go, and it makes me feel quite imbarassed [*sic*] except I realize myself what a great change has really taken place." She discovered to her surprise that "I'm actually growing up as well as out." She grew half an inch in her first six weeks on insulin and wondered, "Isn't that some kind of record, though?" She could hardly wait for her parents to get to Toronto to see for themselves. "I know you will hardly know me as your weak, thin daughter, for I look entirely different everybody says, and I can even see it myself." Insulin was, she wrote, "simply too wonderful for words."

Elizabeth had rarely commented on her appearance during her decline. Now she began to do so regularly. She wrote to her mother that Blanche thought she was "getting to look more like Father everyday, which is very thrilling news for me," and "I simply don't recognize myself as the same person when I look in the mirror." Even so, she didn't want to seem too self-absorbed. "[E]nough about my looks," she exclaimed. "I'll be getting vain if I don't look out, but I was sure you'd be interested to know all the gossip."

The changes in her body were not all positive. The extract contained impurities that caused problems at the injection site.

Elizabeth reported, "my hips are swollen and literally all little lumps all over them now." But she thought it was a small price to pay. "I could put up with absolutely anything to keep on this wonderful diet I'm on now," she told Mrs. Hughes.

Insulin's efficacy remained inconsistent, and that created problems, too. One batch was so weak that Elizabeth had to take as much as five cubic centimeters of it at a time, a challenge considering that the syringe she used contained only two cubic centimeters. Rather than having three injections in her already swollen flesh to deliver the needed amount, Blanche injected her once, left the needle in her ("I feel like a pincushion") while she unscrewed the syringe, and refilled it two more times. This procedure took about 20 minutes and left Elizabeth's leg numb "until I walk on it a bit."

Despite these problems, which she wrote about as mere nuisances, she now felt secure in her future. She finally revealed the confusion of hope and fear with which she had lived. She still was rarely explicit, but her letters included small revelations. She began, without fanfare, to refer to the period before insulin as a time when she was weak. For the first time, she wrote that she was suffering from a "dreadful disease," although she still never referred to it by name. During her decline, her silver watch strap and a gold bracelet had become so loose that she had a jeweler take some links out. Now that she was growing rapidly, these had become tight. She confessed to her mother that she had kept the extra links tucked in a drawer, saving them, "just for this special immergency [*sic*], although I must say I didn't ever expect it to come." And yet she had kept them. Her jewelry had embodied all her private hope for her future.

Many diabetics in this first clinical trial, each in a wretched, depleted state, were brought back from imminent death in what Joslin called "near resurrections." Yet the patients' journeys, while thrilling, came with new sets of problems. Apart from the variation in the quality of insulin, there was much to be learned about how it worked. No one understood how much to use and whether the goal should be to keep the diabetic completely free of showing any sugar in the urine or whether some was all right, and nothing much was known about how and why insulin was working.

Physicians and patients were particularly struggling to understand hypoglycemia, also known as insulin reaction or insulin shock. This phenomenon, identified earlier by Bert Collip, happens when blood sugar falls to a low level because a person has received too much insulin. Diabetics, of course, usually had exactly the opposite problem—blood sugar levels that were too high because their bodies produced no insulin. Doctors and patients now had to find the right amount of insulin to balance the amount of food being eaten. Neither had the knowledge or the technology to calculate this exactly, and so it was unavoidable that diabetics would occasionally experience low blood sugar.

When it happened, the symptoms were frightening and unpleasant. They could begin with a feeling that disaster was imminent, described by one diabetic as like "standing in front of an oncoming train." This was followed by a variety of symptoms that could include profuse sweating, trembling in the muscles, sudden hunger, impaired coordination, accelerated heart rate, and dilated pupils.

Elizabeth experienced many insulin reactions in the first two weeks after Banting began her new diet. She was eating a great deal of food and he prescribed a lot of insulin to match it but with no history to guide either of them, it was trial and error. The episodes were frightening at first, but she quickly became confident about dealing with them and they became fewer and farther apart. Later, when Mrs. Hughes learned and understood more about Elizabeth's treatment, she was worried about her ever being alone in case she experienced a reaction. Elizabeth quickly dismissed this concern: "Listen Mother, I always know when I am having a reaction now because I have had them so much and all I have to do is reach on my table for a kiss [Hershey's chocolate] and then in five minutes I am all right . . . and if one candy didn't seem to be enough for that time why all I'd do would be to eat another one and keep on until I recovered."

After three months, she looked so well and felt so confident that Banting was eager to show her and his high-calorie diet off. He brought in a group of six eminent diabetologists, including Joslin and Allen, to see her. Elizabeth had been nervous about being presented to this tough audience. Joslin was easy, as he was "simply adorable," but she still found Allen intimidating. However, she was able to report home that it was not as bad as she had feared: "Dr. Allen said with his mouth wide open—oh!—and that's all he did. He just kept on saying over and over again that he had never seen such a great change in anyone and he actually cracked a joke as he was leaving saying he was glad to have been introduced to me or he wouldn't have known who it was. Now I think thats [sic] very good of him."

All Joslin could do was "look over at me and smile and say that he never saw anybody with diabetes look so well." So, the meeting with the doctors "went off beautifully."

Elizabeth continued her physical transformation. At the end of November, three and a half months after starting on insulin, she weighed almost 76 pounds "naked." She had gained 30 pounds, more than 65 percent of her body weight.

ELIZABETH BUBBLED WITH newfound energy. The same pleasures that brought her joy when she was wasting away now helped her navigate this exciting new period of her life. A bustling city lay outside her Grosvenor Street apartment and she decided to enjoy it. Beauty and the arts brought her particular pleasure. In Toronto in fall and early winter and without access to a car, she had little opportunity to experience the scenic beauty of Ontario. She and Blanche did get out occasionally to places such as Bond Lake, about 25 miles away at the end of the trolley car line, to see the fall colors, but more commonly they contented themselves with urban pleasures.

She became an avid concertgoer. Toronto in 1922, a city of about a half million people, was bursting with postwar confidence and there was a busy concert program in Massey Hall, which had been built in 1894. The roster of artists Elizabeth heard was dazzling. The season began in earnest in October, and in that month alone she saw Mischa Elman, a Russian-born pianist residing in the United States, whom she loved, and heard the Italian tenor Giulio Crimi. Elizabeth had heard Crimi before and liked him. She especially enjoyed an aria he sang from the opera *La Tosca* that Elizabeth knew well, she reminded her mother, from "the record we have of Caruso singing."

She also heard the Canadian contralto Jeanne Gordon, who was new to Elizabeth. She was a bit more reserved about her out of loyalty to her friend Mme. Louise Homer, whom Gordon had replaced at the Metropolitan Opera. Elizabeth thought Gordon's voice "beautiful" but "I don't think it equals Mme. Homer." Being now 15 years old, Elizabeth was also swayed by Gordon's gown, which she described as "awful," saying that it looked like a "red draperie curtain and clung to her most awfully showing her form in the most hideous manner." However, in the second half of the recital Gordon changed into a costume from *Carmen* for a duet with Crimi. Elizabeth thought she looked "much better," and the audience "went wild" in its appreciation.

That was just the beginning of the musical delights she heard. In one week in November, Elizabeth went to hear the French soprano Emma Calvé and Frieda Hempel, the German-born American singer, performing with the Boston Symphony Orchestra. Elizabeth thought Hempel was "perfectly wonderful" but the *Star* critic was not so kind, describing her condescendingly as "perfect in her way." Later in the month, there was a flurry of great pianists performing in the city. Elizabeth went to see Polish pianist Ignacy Paderewski, who she thought was "too wonderful for words." He came back to play six encores as the audience "cheered and hooted and stamped every time he went offstage." Elizabeth and the *Star* critic were enraptured. A few days later, she went to hear another Polish pianist, Josef Hoffman, who Elizabeth thought was "just as good" as Paderewski. She was transported with delight.

She also went to the cinema, enjoying "several good movies" including *Little Lord Fauntleroy*, based on the book by Frances Hodgson Burnett, which Elizabeth thought was "too sweet for words." She also saw a movie based on another Burnett book, *The Dawn of a Tomorrow*. Additionally, she went to the theater to see the play *Lilian* and the musical of *Daddy Long Legs*, the movie of which she had already seen.

Delightful as these excursions were, they consumed little time compared to the hours she still spent reading, and books continued to be at the center of her world. Once again, she made good use of local public libraries. These had recently been expanded after the city received a gift from one of the charitable foundations of Andrew Carnegie, the industrialist and philanthropist. There were plenty of books from which to choose.

She now picked up Dickens with enthusiasm. Having written to her mother from Bermuda that she enjoyed him, she now gave the lie to that report. "I know you will be surprised and delighted," she told her mother, "when you know I'm beginning to actually adore Dickens." She quickly read *Nicholas Nickleby*, the *Pickwick Papers*, and *Little Dorrit*, finished *Silas Marner* by George Eliot, and continued to find and read books by Hudson.

She also enjoyed her children's magazines. She submitted essays and had three receive special mention in *St. Nicholas* while she was in Toronto, something in which she took great pride. And she still loved reading the adventure stories they offered. When she was missing one issue of *Youth's Companion*, Elizabeth wanted her mother to see "if it isn't lying around down at the State Department somewhere? I hate to miss it for it makes my continued stories sound all crazy." This may not have been a request to which Mrs. Hughes devoted a lot of time.

She also wrote letters, of course, and in them the newly energetic Elizabeth was more forceful about making demands on others. When newlywed sister Catherine failed to write a letter as expected, Elizabeth pouted. "YOU said she was going to write," she complained to her mother, as if Mrs. Hughes were responsible for the actions of her 24-year-old daughter. Elizabeth's own correspondence was prolific. After a month-long pause while her parents were out of the country, her letters home were frequent, all written now on her new portable typewriter. She did not type as carefully as she wrote and made many small errors. She became especially careless with the use of the apostrophe, and occasionally her spelling faltered, too, so she went back over her letters, correcting the mistakes by hand if she found them.

She was now a more confident letter writer to people outside the family but found the writing demands of being in the public eye burdensome. Her fame as a recipient of insulin prompted other diabetics to contact her. "The poor things, I feel so sorry for them," she wrote. But Elizabeth had little inclination to commune with her fellow sufferers and she was in a difficult position. Insulin was still experimental and in short supply but, she wrote, "I suppose I've got to answer," and she did so without any further agonizing.

And she passed on news of friends old and new. Miss Mckay, Blanche's friend in Bermuda, had sent a clipping from the *Royal Gazette* announcing the death in late August of Colonel Alfred Swalm, the U.S. consul in Hamilton who had been so kind to her.

Elizabeth remembered him as "such a sweet man" and immediately wrote a condolence letter to his widow. She passed on to her mother news of another death, this time of someone who was not a friend but who felt like one—"my beloved" William Henry Hudson, whose books brought her so much pleasure.

She knew very few people in Toronto but quickly found some she could visit. Not surprisingly, she spent time with the other two American diabetic children, Teddy Ryder and Ruth Whitehill. They were too young to be real companions to Elizabeth but they saw a lot of each other. This was natural, as they all "had such a common interest and [had been] living so near together." Elizabeth was sad when the children and their families left at the end of September as, she told her mother, "we have become quite fast friends." But as the concert season was just beginning, she did not sit home and pine.

She enjoyed seeing Banting regularly, and occasionally the handsome 23-year-old Charley Best. He had now returned from summer vacation to work on improving insulin production in Toronto. Elizabeth particularly looked forward to his visits, as she had a shy crush on him. She did not meet the other key members of the team. Bert Collip had returned to Alberta for good. Macleod continued to be absorbed by his research on fish insulin and administrative work, particularly as secretary of the university's insulin committee, responsible for resolving its patent and licensing issues.

Despite Banting's routine visits to patients, his life had already changed dramatically since the discovery of insulin. He was in the spotlight, receiving attention from the press and public and fast becoming a celebrity. He no longer lived a hand-to-mouth existence. Instead, he earned a significant salary from the university and Toronto General Hospital, where the specialized diabetes clinic he was to run had opened.

The differences in his life were not just in professional standing. One of his friends, a Dr. Robertson, was horrified when he learned that Banting had met Mrs. Hughes wearing his only, very shabby, suit. He hauled Banting off to a tailor to remedy the situation and simply instructed the tailor to "make this man a suit." Robertson then added an overcoat to the order, chose the fabric, style, and color for both, and even vouched for Banting's ability to pay at some future date.

Banting now dressed better but otherwise had difficulty adjusting to the demands of his newfound fame. His medical colleagues still saw him as difficult and unpredictable, and reporters found him inarticulate. He did a lot of public speaking, but he was never comfortable with it and had to fortify himself with a stiff drink before and afterward. Even though he had all along resented Macleod's ability to stand up and speak easily, he was not comfortable with the reality of what the recognition of the team's accomplishments would bring.

It was hardly surprising, then, that he enjoyed the more simple interactions with his young patients. Banting visited Elizabeth and she enjoyed their conversations. One evening he came to take Elizabeth and Blanche out for a drive, but Blanche was busy, so Elizabeth went alone. He gave her a tour of his office, his rooms, and the labs where insulin was made. She told her mother it was "the most interesting thing I've seen in a long time." Elizabeth was tickled pink, not least because "I felt so grown up going out with a man alone at night!"

Elizabeth was also finding herself something of a local celebrity. Her arrival in Toronto had been front-page news. This was not just because of her father's importance, but because her visit confirmed the importance of the discovery. Insulin was still an unknown quantity and the paper hailed the arrival of "the daughter of the U.S. Secretary of State" as "sufficient proof of its value." But, once settled in, she tried to keep a low public profile. No public officials sought her out to court her for her famous father, as had happened in Bermuda. Toronto was a commercial rather than a political capital. Even so, she was a figure of note.

Elizabeth hated press reports about her. When she told her mother about gaining yet another two pounds, she teased her to "please not let on to a newspaper reporter!" She hated "to be written up like that all over the country" for her own sake, but she also disliked it for Banting's. She thought it was "cheapening to the discovery" but it helped promote people's awareness of the new treatment. Elizabeth was insulin's most famous recipient, and she told her mother that other doctors were teasing Banting "about advertising his discovery through me." She, naively, seems genuinely not to have considered that as a possibility.

However, while people applauded the fact that Elizabeth was "taking the insulin treatment," not everyone thought that the Hugheses were right to leave her in Toronto. During her stay, her parents made only one very brief visit at the end of October. In late November, the *Star* observed that Elizabeth "attracted sympathetic attention" as she "virtually was an exile from her family for more than a year, due to the pressing duties of the father and mother." Even though the family was in contact by letter and telegraph, and radio while the Hugheses were on the high seas, the writers in the Toronto newspapers were unimpressed.

Elizabeth, of course, expressed no such criticism of her parents. She understood the pressures on them and believed her father when he told her in another rare letter that it was "very hard to be a fond father and a Secretary of State at the same time." She continued to appreciate all they did for her. As she realized that she might be "able to live at home and lead a normal life," she told her mother, "I really can never express my gratitude to you and Pa for giving me this wonderful chance!"

SLOWLY, ELIZABETH GRASPED the magnitude of the change that insulin would bring to her life. During her first few weeks on it, not surprisingly, she saw the transformation purely from the point of view of the food she could eat and the changes in her body. But as the weeks passed, she became used to those alterations and her goals became more ambitious.

By early October, she thought she might be so well by the following year that "I'm sure I will be able to do a little studying ... that is a most thrilling thought to me." A few days later, she even contemplated attending school. She felt that "time passes so heavily on my hands. . . . I just long too for some companions my own age again for I've been held back so long, and my brain is fairly dancing around days in order to find something to do." In a true barometer of how far she had come, she observed, "You can't simply read, sew and go to the movies all the time," activities any one of which had been exhausting for her only a few weeks before. She knew that it was "up to you and father to decide the fatal question" and eagerly awaited their answer. She had it merely four days later. They gave their permission for her to go to school in Toronto, and Elizabeth told them she "could almost weep for joy over it."

The next stage on the road to a normal life quickly dawned on her: when she came home to Washington for Christmas she could stay and go to school there rather than in Canada. As she lobbied her parents for this, she hinted at past bitterness about her lonely struggle: "I've realized that theres [sic] no place like home even though you don't always quite realize it at first." She didn't want to stay in Toronto because "I'm definitely sure and positive that I'd be deathly homesick, for I've had to fight that dreadful disease ever since I came into my own so to speak again even though Blanche is here with me."

Elizabeth decided to make her parents feel guilty. Gone was the stoic child and the accommodating tone she had used writing from Bermuda. If she had to stay in Toronto, she wrote, "I'm afraid I should pine away. Especially after having been home for three wonderful weeks at Xmas, and knowing how nice it was and then having to come up here to this place. . . . I don't see how I could do it except perhaps if I could forget that I ever had such a nice home and wonderful ma and pa." Having to come back to Grosvenor Street would even be worse than being at boarding school, because there "you have endless friends and activities to take your thoughts away from home." Elizabeth could "see perfectly clearly what a desperate state I'd be in" and was confident her parents "must appreciate how I feel."

The Hugheses hesitated, but two other developments quickly gave Elizabeth the ammunition she needed to overcome any concern they might have. The first did not concern insulin at all but rather Blanche. Since Elizabeth and Blanche had been in Toronto, Blanche had entered a whirlwind romance and become engaged to be married. One Dr. McClintock had won her heart and Elizabeth completely approved. She thought that he really was "worthy of her" and saw that Blanche was in love. "I was positive of it all the time," she told Mrs. Hughes. "She couldn't have had all the symptons [sic] of it and not have the malady." The couple intended to make their life in California, and Blanche would travel there as soon as she had brought Elizabeth back to Washington for the holidays. So, whatever city Elizabeth would be in, she would need a new nurse.

But things were moving rapidly, and soon Elizabeth reported the next dramatic change. Banting had told her that eight-year-old Ruth, who had returned to Baltimore with her family, now gave herself her own insulin injections. Elizabeth wrote that that news was "altogether too much for me. I was not going to be in any way outdone by a mere girl of eight." So, she made the "bold resolve" to do the same thing. She told her mother the exciting news:

I decided that being captain of my own ship it would be very well for me to manage the target practice every day. So yesterday I resolved to be bold and begin. Thus I cleared the decks thoroughly and myself fired the first shot heard round the world (my world that is). I made a clean breast of it and hit the bulls-eye on the instant causing no ill effect whatever to my target. After shooting all the shells I had, and without the slightest leak whatever in the hold through the force of the concussion, I gave the order to heave to (which I executed myself) and back went the gun and powder all cleaned and ready for further use the next day.

The next day, she was as relaxed about giving herself her shot as if she had been doing it her whole life. Elizabeth was ecstatic and reported that Banting, too, was "tickled to death."

She no longer needed a nurse to do this duty—nor, she realized, did she need one to monitor her food. She could cook her own food and "weigh and figure" quantities, she told her mother. She would even be "perfectly able to live alone (that is if I wanted to) and be well able to do everything for myself. Blanche is elated and so am I, and now things seem to be working out better than ever."

Banting agreed that Elizabeth could easily now take care of herself without any supervision. In late November, Elizabeth launched her last campaign. "You see," she told her mother,

I've lived with this thing from the beginning, and I know every little ins and outs to it and I know just as well as Blanche just what dose to give when I've shown sugar or when I've had a reaction, in fact I've helped B. lots of times deciding. Oh Mothy I don't want anybody, please! You tried me before and I've been true to the game all along and I'll continue to be. I'm not a bit sick or weak any more and I don't want to have somebody watching and hanging around me all the time. . . . Really Mother having not been used to this new treatment, doses, reactions, and all, naturally you are a little worried, but I'm not a bit, for I know all about it, and there's no danger.

She rested her case and the Hugheses folded. Elizabeth was thrilled.

SHE HEADED HOME to begin her life as an insulin-dependent—but independent—diabetic. Her terrible nightmare was over. Before she left Toronto, she sat down to write to her mother what she hoped would be "the last letter I'm going to write you in a very long time." She meant it in a celebratory way. She did not want to be away from home again soon. She explained the plan she and Blanche had devised for adjusting her shots and eating to accommodate the difficulties of the journey and then wished her mother "Goodbye for the last time." She could not wait to be home.

She and Blanche had negotiated their way out of their apartment lease and, on December 1, they boarded a train headed back to Washington. Elizabeth traveled in high spirits. From now on, as she had assured her parents before she left, she was determined to be "absolutely independent" and "Captain of my own ship."

Elizabeth had lived for three years on an average of 800 or fewer calories a day and had done so without retreating into solitude or letting misery overwhelm her. She had lived in the world, seeking solace and distraction in the company of friends. Books had entertained her and allowed her to explore distant lands in her imagination. She had delighted in the beauty of the natural world around her and set goals for herself, enjoying the challenges of writing competitions. She stayed connected to her loving family through a lively correspondence. She always had confidence in her future and never stopped planning for it, even though those plans needed to be adjusted with each setback.

She did not realize that she had been captain of her own ship for a very long time.

CHAPTER 9

I Have Nothing to Complain Of

O N FRIDAY, DECEMBER 1, 1922, seeing the young lady who jumped down onto the platform in Union Station in Washington, D.C., must have been a dream come true for the Hugheses. Her hair was shining, her eyes were bright, and although still small for her 15 years—barely five feet tall and only 75 pounds—Elizabeth was bursting with energy. Considering the emaciated, 48-pound child they had greeted five months earlier after her return from Bermuda, her parents must have been barely able to contain their joy and amazement.

For the moment, though, there was no time to consider the momentous change. There was a flurry of activity on the platform while all the bags and baggage of the new Elizabeth were safely taken off the train. She had warned her mother that she had accumulated a lot during her more than three months in Toronto: "3 trunks, a hatbox, 2 suitcases, and a bag, plus my typewriter," as well as a package with some craft work she was doing. And that did not include any of Blanche's things.

Fortunately, there were porters to do the heavy lifting and they all arrived home in high spirits, ready to exchange their news. The time of their arrival was perfect. It was the day after Thanksgiving. The holiday offered a brief break in the Hugheses' busy schedule, and they had a weekend to gaze at their transformed daughter.

Once home, Elizabeth had another treat to anticipate. Mrs. Hughes had arranged for her older daughter, Catherine, and son-in-law, Chauncey Waddell, to come down to Washington from New York for Christmas so the sisters could meet again. They had not seen each other since Elizabeth had gone to Bermuda the previous December. Not only had Elizabeth's life changed dramatically since then, but Catherine's had, too, since she had married and moved permanently to New York. The sisters had a lot to celebrate. Mrs. Hughes was paying for the newlyweds to travel down as a present to them, but as Elizabeth told her mother, "it will be just as much of a Christmas present for me."

But before Catherine and Chauncey arrived, there was an important farewell to make. Elizabeth had to say good-bye to Blanche. The two had spent three years in close companionship. At first Blanche had been the disciplinarian, but the relationship changed as Elizabeth matured and grew in confidence. While Elizabeth wasted away, Blanche had been her caregiver and her friend. In Toronto, as her energy returned, they had enjoyed city life, both eager for concerts and plays, and had shared a bed in their tiny apartment, huddling together for warmth as snow fell outside. Now Elizabeth felt secure managing her own treatment and no longer needed her nurse's advice. Blanche also had a new life ahead of her, as she was soon to marry and move to California. The two parted and never met again.

Elizabeth quickly reclaimed the life she had longed for. After the holidays she started attending Miss Madiera's School, then just off Dupont Circle, barely a five-minute walk from her home. There, Elizabeth found an intimate setting where she could catch up on what she had missed, be challenged, and excel.

She made new friends and got together with old ones. Even though a blossoming teenager, she was still too young to be part of her parents' social world. But she did not stay home studying all the time; she had her own social engagements. Her return to society was signaled when a formal portrait photograph of her appeared in the *Post* in March 1923. She was now available for tennis parties, horseback-riding expeditions, and concert invitations.

However, life was not all smooth sailing for the Hughes family. President Harding died in August that year and Vice President Calvin Coolidge assumed the presidency. Mr. Hughes had to work within a new administration. Fortunately, after a tumultuous few weeks as the reins of government changed hands, he had no difficulty adjusting to the new president.

Elizabeth's new life on insulin also had its challenges. At first, things went well. Just over six weeks after her return to Washington, she wrote Frederick Banting to tell him that "I have grown one half an inch in a months time." But the speed of this and other changes in her body was unsettling. At the beginning of January 1923, she reported she weighed "84¾ pounds," nearly

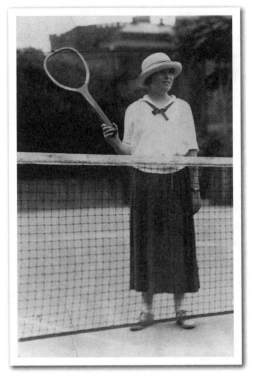

Elizabeth on the tennis court, circa 1923.
Courtesy Library of Congress.

double her weight of late summer. No matter how necessary
for health, her new body felt strange. She told Banting she was
already "trying to get in some real strenuous exercise everyday
in order to work off some of my calories, and also to prevent
gaining so much." She started swimming and horseback riding.
A couple of weeks later, she weighed a mere 92 pounds but now
thought it was time to reduce her diet: "I don't want to gain so
very fast the way I was doing, and yet I don't want to lose any
so I hope I can strike a happy medium in this way."

Despite these anxieties, she told him that she was pleased to take on "a much hardier look" and develop muscle tone through her regular exercise. She was able to adjust her diet and insulin when she was sick. "Insulin doesn't work the same with a fever," she reported. But the quality of insulin could still vary and she had trouble figuring out exactly how much to eat for her stage of life. A year later, in early 1924, she weighed 103 pounds, and now told Banting she was worried that she "did not seem to be growing or developing in accord with my age." She began to increase the amount of food she was eating but, for the time being, a steady, healthy weight eluded her.

She had a more severe setback that summer. She became ill and could not find the right balance between insulin and food. She went to stay at Frederick Allen's clinic for a month. At the time, her parents were in London for an American Bar Association meeting (Mr. Hughes was president of the organization that year), and Elizabeth had been staying with Catherine and Chauncey in New York when she was taken ill. However, this difficulty was soon behind her and by September she was back in Washington with her parents, joining her contemporaries in sports. She played in an annual tennis tournament for the diplomatic community. This was hosted by Mary Henderson, an important Washington society hostess and wife of Senator John Henderson of Missouri, at their mansion, Henderson's Castle.

Elizabeth now took Washington high society in stride. Mrs. Coolidge invited her to join a White House "musicale" at which the Russian-born pianist Sergei Rachmaninoff played. She went to hear the New York Symphony perform with her mother; Helen Taft, wife of former President William Howard Taft, who since 1921 was chief justice of the Supreme Court; and Lady Isabella Howard, wife of the British ambassador. All were sitting in the theater box of Mabel Boardman, the secretary of the American Red Cross.

Only on rare occasions was Elizabeth unsure how to handle herself. One day, while strolling in Washington, she met Chief Justice Taft, who chatted to her as they walked along. But she was uncomfortable. She knew Mrs. Taft better and was not so relaxed with the former president. Additionally, when she walked with her father, they did so in silence, as she knew he was absorbed with work. She was sure Taft was just making conversation because convention required it. As she later recalled, she decided to put him at his ease. "Mr. Chief Justice," she said, "you don't need to talk to me." Taft thought this line was hilarious and later telephoned Mr. Hughes to repeat it and share the joke.

Elizabeth had begun to put her terrible years of starvation behind her. But in 1925, two changes occurred that gave her the opportunity to revisit the places where she had spent so many of her declining months. The first concerned her parents. With Coolidge's election victory in November 1924, Mr. Hughes felt it was time to bow out of public life and tendered his resignation as secretary of state. He wanted to reclaim his privacy and return to his lucrative New York law practice to restore the family's wealth, which years of public service had drained. Mrs. Hughes was also eager to give up the relentless rounds of entertaining and return to a more tranquil existence.

Did Elizabeth resent the fact that now, when her crisis was

past, her parents decided to step away from their public duties, be more available to her, and live a more restful life? There is no hint that she did. She was still immensely proud of them and celebrated their accomplishments. She later remembered that, at this time, she was determined to put her terrible years behind her and her parents "agreed to forget the diabetes with her."

The second change involved Elizabeth directly. At the end of February, she graduated from high school and confided in her diary "how I do hate to say 'goodbye' to everyone." But adventure beckoned. Before the family moved back to New York, Mr. and Mrs. Hughes and Elizabeth would spend three months in Bermuda, which their good friend Mrs. Hamlin helped them arrange, and another three at Lake George. Elizabeth would be retracing the journeys of her starving years.

In early March 1925, as soon as the new administration was sworn in, they left on their travels. There had been fond farewells between the Hugheses and the Washington political community. At the last two "at home" teas that her mother hosted, Elizabeth counted more than 1,100 people attending in total. When she and her parents boarded the train to leave Washington, many members of the new cabinet and the diplomatic corps were there to say good-bye. Elizabeth would miss this world, but she eagerly anticipated the journeys ahead of her.

Once in Bermuda, her days were not completely frivolous. She had to spend hours working for her father, helping him keep up with his voluminous correspondence and speech writing. On many fine Bermudian mornings, her diary entries noted simply "typewrite and receive dictation." She still read a great deal, but on this trip usually only when there was no livelier pursuit on offer. Most afternoons, she rode her bike or played tennis with other young people. One day she enjoyed walking around Honeymoon Cottage, where she and Blanche had lived for six months. She met up with some of the same families she had seen before and saw her good friend Connie McLane. Mrs. Hamlin's daughter Anna was also there. Anna was about seven years older than Elizabeth, and on her previous visit, the young woman's world of parties and tennis had no appeal for Elizabeth. Nor had Elizabeth's quiet world of reading and the contemplation of nature appealed to Anna, and the two had rarely socialized. But now with Elizabeth full of energy, Anna swept Elizabeth up in her world, and the two played tennis and went to the garrison band concerts together.

But in April 1925, tragedy struck. Anna fell ill. She suffered again from what Elizabeth called her "old malady." This was peritonitis, resulting from an intestinal rupture that occurred when the mesenteric artery that supplies blood to the intestines became blocked. When it occurred four years earlier, Anna had barely survived. Elizabeth could imagine the pain she was in. "Oh dear, I feel so sorry for A," she commented in her diary. Anna had two surgeries in quick succession at the hospital in Hamilton, but Elizabeth knew the second was a "last resort" and that there was really "no hope." The young woman's parents had already been summoned by telegraph, but they did not arrive in time. Anna died at age 24. Elizabeth was deeply moved. After Anna's body was laid out, she went to see her and confided in her diary that she "looked lovely, but the ghastly suffering & pain she went through showed in her face."

Elizabeth and Mr. and Mrs. Hughes joined the Hamlins and a few others in a small service. The Hugheses must have been filled with compassion for their friends. It had only been five years earlier that they had buried their eldest daughter, Helen, and it was only three since they had come close to losing Elizabeth. Their youngest had never known just how desperate her situation was. But the next day, Elizabeth felt the need for solace. She went over to Honeymoon Cottage again and walked in the neighborhood that had once been a favorite.

By early June the Hughes family was back in the United States, renting a home at Lake George. Elizabeth continued to do secretarial work for her father, swim, and play tennis. And there were Hoopes, Hydes, and Homers to visit. She spent hours with her good friend Polly Hoopes, chatted with whichever of the Homer twins was available, and of course saw Mme. Homer, who, she noted in her diary, was "just as sweet" as ever. Elizabeth passed her driving test in Glens Falls, and her parents gave her an early birthday present: a new small touring car, an Essex. "Oh boy," she exclaimed in her diary, "at last my dream has come true."

At the end of the summer, Elizabeth was setting off on another adventure: college. Elizabeth had applied to Barnard, the women's college affiliated with and next to Columbia University in New York. When she received her acceptance letter, she sent up "three cheers" in her diary. She was impressed by the "nice atmosphere up there" and wanted to be able to stay with her parents in the family's new apartment at 1020 Fifth Avenue, at East 83rd Street. By late September, she had registered and begun her classes. Only a few short years before, she could not have imagined being part of this world. Now here she was. Not surprisingly, she loved it.

THE DISCOVERERS OF insulin had an equally exciting couple of years. Fame, glory, and prizes were heaped on them, but bad feeling and bitterness among them detracted from the pleasure of those rewards. Of course, there had occasionally been tension between Banting and John Macleod and Banting and Bert Collip before, and these burst into the open again when the discoverers won the Nobel Prize in Medicine in 1923. That should have been a cause for celebration, but Banting was furious when he heard that the Nobel committee had awarded it to himself and Macleod alone. At first, he threatened to refuse the prize and stormed around "helling and damning," according to one observer. Then he decided to share his prize with Charlie Best. Best, enjoying his celebrity, was, at that moment, giving a lecture to Harvard medical students in Boston. Banting sent a telegram to Elliott Joslin, who was in the audience, for him to read aloud to the crowd: "I ascribe to Best equal share in the discovery stop hurt that he is not acknowledged by Nobel trustees stop will share with him."

Elliott Joslin later remembered that day. He particularly recalled that many students were present. Best's participation in the research that led to the discovery had changed the status of students everywhere. They all now saw their potential to play major roles in research. Best, after all, was still one of them. They were sitting in every nook and cranny, Joslin remembered, even hanging "over the rails at the back of the high auditorium." The former president of Harvard, Charles Elliot, was sitting in the front row and when Joslin received Banting's telegram, Joslin passed it to Elliot to read out to the crowd. The announcement resulted in "pandemonium."

A few days later, Macleod announced that he would split some of his share of the prize with Collip, but this move did not mollify Banting. He and some other researchers thought about writing to the Nobel committee to protest Macleod's award more vigorously. Banting thought that Macleod did not deserve this honor for what he saw as his minor role in the team's accomplishments. But, ultimately, for the sake of Canada (they were the nation's first Nobel laureates), honor, and good manners, they were encouraged to put down their pens.

However, debate in the scientific community as to who should have received recognition for the discovery simmered on. That argument was not focused on the personalities of the Toronto group; rather, it was the many researchers who had toiled in the field for years and their partisans who were upset. The Romanian Nicolas Paulesco and American Israel Kleiner had insulin in their pancreatic extracts but had not been able to purify them enough to get effective results. Some argued that there had been a process of discovery rather than a moment, and that the Toronto team had simply expanded and refined existing knowledge. If indeed there was a moment, it was probably when Collip was able to produce a more pure, nontoxic version of the extract in January 1922. It would have been only a matter of time before someone else had managed to do this. But the Toronto team was first, saving the lives of many grateful people, including Elizabeth Hughes.

The Nobel committee made the unusual decision to award

the prize to Banting and Macleod the first time they were nominated. More commonly, people were nominated multiple times before receiving the prize. But as the nominating letter by scientist and Nobel laureate August Krogh argued, it was a momentous discovery of "both theoretical and practical importance." The committee then tried to find the best choice of whom to recognize for that accomplishment and settled on Banting and Macleod.

Banting was not easily able to move on from these exciting years and had no research success thereafter. He flitted about from topic to topic, finding little that gripped him but feeling enormous public pressure to achieve something else after his youthful burst of glory. Despite this, his public stature stayed high and honors poured in. The Canadian government voted him a lifelong annuity. The Royal Society of Canada and the Canadian Medical Association awarded him medals. He became a fellow of the British Royal College of Surgeons and finally in 1934 was knighted, becoming Sir Frederick Banting, a title he never used. He became and remained an important public figure.

However, Banting found himself on the front pages of the newspapers for other reasons: his two marriages—neither to his former fiancée, Edith Roach—and his one sensational divorce. He and Edith made each other unhappy with their on again–off again relationship for a couple of years before they finally parted in 1924. Later that same year, he met and quickly married Marion Robertson, an X-ray technician at Toronto General Hospital. They made each other miserable. Their divorce case in 1931–32, with its mutual accusations of marital misconduct, regularly made the front pages of the Toronto papers. Each side fanned the flames until, finally, Marion's father joined the fray. In an era of public discretion about such things, the *Star* reported that Mr. Robertson had named a woman in court, Miss Blodwen Davies, whom he claimed Banting had "spent many hours alone with." That brought matters to a swift conclusion. The divorce was finalized and the scandal died down. Banting and Blodwen severed their relationship shortly thereafter. In 1938, Banting met Henrietta Ball, almost 20 years his junior, and they married a year later. When war broke out in September 1939, Banting again enlisted in the Royal Canadian Army Medical Corps. He was killed on a military flight to England in February 1941 when his plane crashed in Newfoundland.

His former mentor and later rival, John Macleod, continued to work at the University of Toronto for several years after the discovery. He wrote several books on diabetes and insulin, lobbied for international standards for insulin production, and monitored the university's patent interests in the drug. In 1927, he returned to his native Scotland to an appointment at the University of Aberdeen, where he enjoyed new teaching and research responsibilities. Crippling arthritis cut short his work before he died in 1935.

Charley Best had a longer and happier life. He married Margaret Mahon and, two years after sharing the Nobel Prize, graduated at the top of his class from medical school. He and Margaret traveled to London, where he did postgraduate research, completed a doctorate in science at the University of London (in Britain awarded for a sustained contribution to knowledge), and returned to Canada to take over Macleod's position at the University of Toronto. There, among his other accomplishments, he supervised a team that began to work on heparin, a blood anticoagulant. It had been isolated in 1916 by researchers at John Hopkins University, but they had found it to be toxic and expensive to produce. By 1935, Best's group found a way to purify heparin, which is still used today in many surgeries. He went on to serve in World War II, becoming director of medical research for the Royal Canadian Navy. After the war he turned his attention back to diabetes, especially educational programs, continued with his research, and traveled extensively lecturing.

In his later years, Best reminisced about the discovery. He was reluctant to criticize Macleod because of a "residual loyalty to his memory" and the fact that there was much that Best found "fair" about Macleod's accounts of the events of that tumultuous year. Yet he felt that much of the tension within the group lay at Macleod's door. He had chosen to "dominate rather than lead" the team. "It wasn't the way to do it," Best thought. There were ways they could have moved forward without conflict. It was, he remembered, "a difficult situation for two junior people [himself and Banting] to counteract." Honors were also heaped on Best as the years passed, and he participated in great international celebrations to mark the 50th anniversary of the discovery of insulin. He died six years later, in 1978.

Bert Collip also went on to accomplish more in the world of research. He returned to Alberta, where he was hailed as a hero, but he did not rest on his laurels. He added a medical degree to his PhD and, while getting that, conducted considerable research in endocrinology. After five years, he was offered a job at McGill University in Montreal and he, his wife, Ray, and their growing family relocated there. During his years at that institution, he helped turn McGill into a great research center. He and his fellow researchers made landmark discoveries concerning placental and pituitary hormones.

Collip and Banting later buried their differences and became friends. They served together on the National Research Council that Banting chaired. Just before Banting's fateful flight, he visited Collip in Montreal. Indeed, Collip was one of the last people to see Banting alive, a fitting end after the ways their lives had intertwined. Collip himself also had distinguished wartime medical service, joining the Royal Canadian Army Medical Corps and organizing naval and aviation medical research. After the war he moved on to the University of Western Ontario in London, where he also developed a medical research program. He died from a stroke in 1965.

Frederick Allen and Elliott Joslin, two famous prediscovery diabetes specialists, also traveled divergent paths after insulin. Allen's group of patients who received insulin in that first clinical trial that began in August 1922 represented the largest single cohort to be studied, and his meticulous records served well those studying the effects of the new drug. As the years passed, he turned his attention elsewhere. He experimented in hypertension and was one of the first to recommend a low-salt diet.

But life did not go well for him. Allen had never been a good businessman, and bad investments and the stock market crash of 1929 led him to close the clinic. Although he received the Banting medal from the American Diabetes Association in 1949 for his contributions to diabetic research, he was bitter that the glories of the discovery belonged to others. He lived to old age but never found another project to engage him or to offer him the respect and success he had once enjoyed. In his eighties, he was still experimenting, this time in cancer research, but doing so alone, in the basement of the Pondville State Hospital in Massachusetts. He died in 1964, and even though he had been stern, taciturn, and socially awkward, his friends remembered that he had the capacity for great kindness toward his patients and those who worked for him.

Joslin, in contrast, thrived in the post-insulin world. He recognized that the discovery simply ended one phase of people's experience with diabetes. He expanded his Boston clinic and transformed it into a center for the treatment of and research into the new problems that were appearing as people lived with diabetes for many years. These were complications such as increased incidence of heart disease, loss of kidney function, circulation problems, nerve and eye damage, and women experiencing difficulties carrying pregnancies to term. Joslin became good friends with Best. Apart from their mutual interest in diabetes, the two shared a love of horseback riding and rode whenever they got together. After Joslin died in 1962, Best wrote that he and Banting had "loved him" for his skill and knowledge, "his unselfishness, and his charm." The Joslin Diabetes Foundation took over Joslin's work and today, under the name of the Joslin Diabetes Center, it remains a center of diabetic research, clinical care, and education.

THE FATE OF ALL those associated with the discovery of diabetes was far from Elizabeth's mind as she enjoyed the delights of college. She played sports, went to movies, the theater, concerts, and dances, had lunch with friends—and attended classes. She did well, enjoying her history and French classes and participating in the history club.

Not surprisingly, she also was active in politics. She worked on the New York gubernatorial campaign of 1926 for Ogden Mills, the Republican candidate who lost badly to Democratic governor Al Smith. In her diary entry, she was philosophical: "Such is life—we shouldn't cry over spilled milk." She had a more satisfying experience in 1928, when she was an organizer of a Hoover for President Club that had a vigorous campaign on campus to bring out the vote for its candidate. She had the pleasure of being part of Hoover's landslide victory. It was, she noted in her diary, "Thrills & thrills & thrills!" Elizabeth did not entirely devote herself to politics that year. She was also on the organizing committee of the Barnard Junior Prom. She loved the big evening, staying up dancing until 3:30 A.M. and then going out for breakfast. She confided in her diary that she had "never had such a good time."

She still struggled to find a comfortable weight. She was unhappy when she shot up to 158 pounds during her first year at Barnard. She decided that was too much for her now approximately five-foot-three-inch frame. Slowly, she adjusted to student life and lost the 20 pounds or so she had gained. Finally, her weight steadied, although she occasionally fasted to fit into a dress she wanted to wear. By the time she left college, she had found a balance between eating, exercise, and insulin and a daily routine that she maintained for the rest of her life.

During her college years, with her parents now free to travel, Elizabeth spent each summer with them, going to some of the places she had previously only read about. In the summer of 1926, accompanied by Polly Hoopes, the Hugheses traveled to France, England, Scotland, and Italy. The following year they went again, this time with a college friend, another Elizabeth, traveling through France to the Pyrenees Mountains and the Riviera. The following year, Elizabeth went again with her parents and a college friend, Clara, to central Europe, visiting Berlin, Dresden, Vienna, and Prague before heading into Switzerland.

While in Berlin, Elizabeth had a chance to fulfill another childhood dream. She and her father went up for a joyride in a plane. Elizabeth found it terrifying, something Mr. Hughes thought funny, probably remembering her letters from Lake George begging for permission to fly. With maturity, she had lost the stomach for spills and thrills.

The years 1929 and 1930 may have been difficult ones for the nation as the economy collapsed, but they were fine ones for the Hughes family and great ones for Elizabeth. In spring 1929, she graduated from college. Shortly thereafter, her father took up an appointment as a justice at the world court in The Hague in the Netherlands, and Elizabeth joined her parents there for the whole summer. That year, her brother, Charles, was appointed solicitor general and, in November, Elizabeth's boyfriend, William T. Gossett, a young lawyer in her father's firm, proposed. It was, she told her diary, "the happiest day of my life."

There was one snag. Even though she and Bill had been dating seriously for months, she had not yet told him about her diabetes. She was in a state of "bliss" according to her diary, so it took her a couple of weeks to pluck up the courage. In early December, she told her mother about their engagement and she was "tickled to death." But Elizabeth still had not had the necessary conversation with Bill. It was critical. Apart from him needing to know about the occasional insulin reaction she might have, he also had to be told that it might not be possible for them to have a family. Before insulin, diabetic women were usually unable to carry pregnancies to term, and few successfully had done so in the few years since. She wasted no more time. The next evening, she simply recorded in her diary that she and Bill "hash [talk] desperately." Elizabeth need not have worried. The wedding was still on.

Their marriage in December 1930 marked the end of a banner year. It had begun with a great honor. When Taft stepped down as chief justice of the Supreme Court, Charles Evans Hughes was nominated to replace him. His son, Charles, then gave him a great gift, resigning his own position as solicitor general so that his father could accept the appointment without any conflict of interest. In February 1930, Elizabeth watched with pride as her father was sworn in to begin the last and most distinguished phase of his long career.

Elizabeth and Bill would make their home in the New York area, but first she relocated to Washington with her parents to their new home on R Street, near Sheridan Circle in Kalorama Heights, close to their old neighborhood. They were married in that house in a quiet, small ceremony in late December. She knew that stress was not good for her, so she did not want a grand affair like Catherine's wedding or even a more modest one like her brother's had been. That did not mean that the weeks before were calm. She had, as the *Washington Post* reported, a "wide acquaintance among the younger set in Washington." That meant there was a flurry of celebratory teas and lunches—including one at the White House, hosted by Mrs. Hoover. There was shopping to be done for her wedding trousseau and letters of thanks to be written for the armloads of presents that were arriving at the house.

It was a hectic time, but the wedding day itself was easy. It was a Hughes family affair. Bill Gossett's parents could not attend because his mother was ill, and Catherine and Chauncey were abroad. Only Elizabeth's parents and her brother, Charlie, and his family were there. The child who had been near death eight years earlier was now a healthy young woman and a glowing bride. As befitting the private occasion, she did not wear a formal wedding gown. Rather, the *Post* reported, she wore "an afternoon gown of velvet trimmed with ermine and a corsage bouquet of gardenias. She had no attendants." After the wedding breakfast, the couple left for a honeymoon trip to Elizabeth's beloved Bermuda. It was, she told her diary, "the best year yet!!!!!!"

CHARLES EVANS HUGHES served on the court for 11 years, handing down some landmark decisions on Franklin Delano Roosevelt's New Deal legislation after Roosevelt was elected to the presidency in 1932. Hughes opposed the president's attempt to pack the court and sided with the majority in striking down the National Industrial Recovery Act, although he sided with Roosevelt on other New Deal legislation. Hughes stepped down from the court in 1941 when his health began to decline. Meanwhile, Mrs. Hughes enjoyed the quieter life that had begun in 1925 when she left the public stage. Between then and her death in 1945, she guarded her privacy carefully. The public Antoinette Hughes was someone who, her obituary writers observed, had a "congenial manner" but was more noted for "the seclusion she had managed to preserve."

Her family remembered her differently. She may indeed have rarely held leading roles in any organization, but she was not without strong opinions. In 1940, through her lifelong membership in the Daughters of the American Revolution, she and her husband sponsored the performance of the African American contralto Marion Anderson at the Lincoln Memorial in Washington, D.C. The DAR had refused Anderson permission to perform in Constitution Hall, owned by the organization, because she was black. Led by Eleanor Roosevelt, some outraged members of the DAR, opera lovers, and supporters of racial justice quickly organized the replacement venue. Antoinette Hughes was all three, and she sponsored the new concert "with pleasure." But this was a rare step. She much preferred to be in the background in matters of public policy.

To her family, she was the glue that held them all together. She kept in close contact with all her children and their families. Her bond to her husband was as strong at the end of their marriage as it had been at the beginning. They wrote each other love poems to mark anniversaries and birthdays, and she told her "darling husband" a few years before her death that he had been "all in all to me." A year later on their wedding anniversary, he wrote to her: "I love you more than ever—though that hardly seems possible." He and her children, including

Elizabeth, were at her side when she died. Mr. Hughes survived three short years without her.

The men in the family, Bill Gossett, Chauncey Waddell, and Charles Hughes Jr., were the executors of the Hughes estate. Despite this, Elizabeth went through her father's papers before they were given to the Library of Congress. She removed from them anything that referred to her diabetes and destroyed all photographs of herself from the time of her crisis. She was determined that that part of her life would not be a matter of public record. Before his death, her father had been interviewed by his biographer, Marlo Pusey, and Mr. Hughes had preserved Elizabeth's privacy and not revealed anything about her illness. Thus, Pusey's prize-winning biography of Mr. Hughes's life and work that came out in 1951 contained no mention of it. Elizabeth was determined that no one should know of her condition. If anyone vaguely remembered reports of her illness in the press, she told them they were thinking of her sister, Helen, who had died in 1920.

Not all of Frederick Banting's first patients closed down that chapter of their lives so firmly. Others stayed in touch with Banting, seeing him regularly. Teddy Ryder, who had been a small boy when he and Elizabeth were in Toronto, continued to live at home, and the family visited Banting whenever they were in Toronto. Jim Havens of Rochester, who had been sent trial batches of insulin on the train in the spring of 1922, also maintained a pleasant relationship with Banting. After he had been on insulin a couple of years, he sent Banting a photograph of "your boy Jim" (himself) skiing. Following his marriage in 1927, he and his wife, and later with children in tow, used to camp in Ontario and always visited Banting on their way home. Decades later, Jim admitted to Joslin that "[p]art of me certainly went away when Fred Banting was lost in Newfoundland!"

Jim Havens went on to have a rich life. He had started drawing to pass the time when he was living on the Allen plan and later taught himself printmaking. He became accomplished in that art, making both linoleum cuts and woodcuts, and was elected to the National Academy of Design. His works are in the collections of the New York Public Library and the Metropolitan Museum of Art in New York City. Although he was beginning to experience some hints of complications connected to diabetes later in life, his death in 1960 was attributed to colon cancer.

In contrast, Elizabeth shut the door on her starving years, even their happy conclusion, and brought a veil of silence down on her illness. After a brief flurry of correspondence with Banting following her return to Washington, a summer visit from him when he was in Washington later that year, and a note she sent to congratulate him on winning the Nobel Prize in Medicine ("you certainly deserve the highest possible honor they can give you"), their contact slowly ended. After she had left high school, she told him she had stopped weighing her food and had found that she could do just as well by "approximating"—something she found liberating and "a great relief." Her last letter to Banting was from college her sophomore year. She updated him on some of her college activities and told him, "I feel just wonderfully and am very happy in my work, so you see I have nothing to complain of."

She never contacted him again. In 1980, more than 50 years later, historian Michael Bliss tracked Elizabeth down to interview her for the book he was writing about the discovery of insulin. The interview was, of course, mostly Bliss asking her questions about her time in Toronto. But Elizabeth asked him one: "What ever happened to dear Dr. Banting?" Bliss filled her in.

Elizabeth repeatedly described to Bliss her time enduring starvation therapy as a nightmare. Even thinking of the little scale on which Blanche had weighed every crumb of food "drives me crazy," she admitted. "In order to put it out of my mind, I had to sever all connection with it." Only her husband, Bill, and one or two lifelong friends, such as Polly Hoopes Beeman, knew about her illness; she otherwise told no one. She kept disciplined eating habits, regular mealtimes, and a strict regimen of daily exercise. She took her two shots a day discreetly. The first one of the day she could easily do as part of her morning routine. For the second, she went into her bedroom at five P.M. and closed the door. Her children saw nothing unusual in this and did not learn of her condition until they were adults.

After the excitement of the discovery and her deliverance from a terrible existence, Elizabeth moved on with her life.

DESPITE THIS, SHE KEPT herself informed about diabetic research. For some time, she knew that she was one of the lucky ones. Rural physicians or those who were not sophisticated about adapting to radical new treatments only slowly accepted insulin. For years, stories appeared in professional journals, such as *Hygeia,* published by the American Medical Association, encouraging physicians to be open to using insulin and affirming "diabetes may now be controlled in the home." Additionally, since no private or public medical insurance existed yet, its cost was beyond the means of many. To remedy that, some philanthropists formed groups to raise money to provide insulin to the poor. One in New York, which Elizabeth's brother, Charles, joined, was the Insulin Committee, which included the financier and philanthropist Felix M. Warburg and Marshall Field III, heir to the department store fortune. This committee's initial donor list included some of the city's wealthiest families. Still, it would take years for knowledge of insulin to be fully disseminated and its benefits generally available.

Elizabeth knew that having children would be risky, but she was determined. And with the help of her physician and her own rigid discipline, she gave birth to three children. The first, in 1934, was Antoinette (Tonie) Carter ("She is so adorable & I can hardly believe she is ours and it all isn't a dream"), followed by W. Thomas Jr. and Elizabeth Evans. Each was delivered by cesarean section and she miscarried only once, between her second and third children.

Elizabeth and Bill Gossett's life together embodied much of the Hughes ethos. They committed themselves to their family, work, and an array of public service and philanthropic endeavors. Making their home first in Bronxville, New York, and then in Bloomfield Hills, Michigan, after Bill became general counsel and vice president of Ford Motor Company, public service was central to their lives. Elizabeth was active in the Junior League and American Red Cross in Bronxville. But once they moved to Detroit, education and racial justice became the common threads of their service. Elizabeth sat on

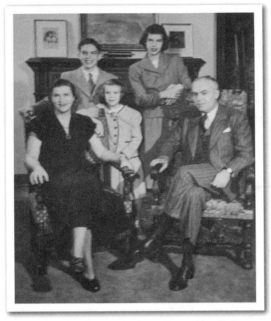

The Gossett family, 1948. Courtesy Gossett Family Papers.

the board of her children's school, Kingswood in Cranbrook, Michigan, and became a trustee of Barnard College in 1957. She was a key agent in establishing Oakland University in Rochester, Michigan, initially known as Michigan State University–Oakland. William Gossett became a leading board member and fundraiser for the United Negro College Fund, serving as chairman of that organization from 1961 to 1967. In the racial turbulence at the end of the 1960s, Elizabeth and her husband co-chaired a new Committee for Commitment to Brotherhood organized jointly by the National Conference of Christians and Jews, the Urban League, the National Association for the Advancement of Colored People, and the Southern

Christian Leadership Conference. Separately and together, public service was a defining feature of their lives.

As Elizabeth matured, she continued to savor many of the joys that had sustained her in her crisis. Music was an ongoing passion. She attended every opera performance she could get to in either Detroit or New York, taking particular pleasure in Richard Wagner's *Götterdämmerung* and *Tristan and Isolde*. She also enjoyed attending the Detroit Symphony and sat on its board of directors for many years. She continued to read voraciously, enjoying newspapers, magazines, biographies, and novels. Her son, Tom, remembers her "'purring' seated in her favorite chair." She continued to read travel literature but augmented it with yet more travel, returning to Europe and adding South America and China to her destinations. She still enjoyed social activity, made and kept up with friends all over the world, and was, like her mother, a "consummate hostess" who enjoyed throwing large, elegant parties. Flowers and nature, and her homegrown tomatoes, brought her pleasure, but the passion for it gave way to other interests. She came to love golf, which she and her husband played on summer weekends. She was an avid baseball fan, supporting the Brooklyn Dodgers as long as she lived in New York and then, after moving to Detroit, switching her support to the Tigers. A summer's day would find her, her son remembers, listening to games "on a radio turned up full volume—the sounds drifting out through the windows flung open in Mother's bedroom."

Elizabeth never became the writer she had dreamed she would. However, she put her pen to the service of the many organizations with which she volunteered. One of these was the Supreme Court Historical Society. In 1974, she was instrumental in founding this society dedicated to honoring the legacy of the court and its justices. She served as its first president. Two years later, to celebrate her father's memory, she wrote an article about him that was published in the society's yearbook. Fifty years after her triumphs in *St. Nicholas,* she again saw something she wrote in print.

Elizabeth Evan Hughes Gossett died in April 1981. She had given permission for her story to be made public after her death. She did not live to know of some great changes in the treatment of diabetes: the introduction of human insulin, synthetically created by geneticists; the advent of small, portable electronic devices that provided fast, accurate measurements of blood sugar from just a pinprick of blood; the introduction of small insulin pumps that allow some diabetics to dispense with injections by delivering insulin into the body 24 hours a day; transplants of islets of Langerhans; or the possibility of creating new islets using stem cells.

But despite these great advances in knowledge and treatment, the experience of diabetics remains, in the words of physician and historian Chris Feudtner, "bittersweet." The sweetness, of course, is that diabetics no longer have to endure starvation therapy and face certain death. The bitterness is that an insulin-dependent diabetic's life is still one of strict dietary control and requires what some feel is an oppressive regime of care and regularity. And while close dietary management and exercise can significantly reduce the risk of complications, it is sometimes not enough.

For Elizabeth, bitterness, when she felt it, was not an emotion that stayed with her for long. Insulin released her from a prison so terrible that for most of her life she could not bear to talk about it, yet she had lived those years with determination, grace, and hope.

Following her death, when her friends and family gathered to celebrate her life, she was remembered for her public service and her character. One eulogist noted particularly her "avid pursuit of self directed scholarship and perpetual inquiry" and considered her "a model of enlightened individual responsibility for self-improvement and personal growth." The speaker, a dean of Oakland University, never knew that the qualities he was celebrating may well have saved her life.

Elizabeth Evans Hughes was diagnosed with a fatal disease. But she was lucky. She was born at the right time, in the right place, and to a well-connected family. Still, it was neither her luck nor her disease that defined her. It was always her love of learning; her delight in nature, music, and art; her love of writing; a commitment to her family and community; and her desire to stay involved in a meaningful way with the world around her.

Throughout her life, privacy about her diabetes was critical to her. She was afraid that if others knew the gravity of her illness they would fuss over her, offer her unsolicited advice, or ask prying questions. Yet she was a compassionate woman, and she realized toward the end of her life that hers was a story that others might want to know. Books had helped sustain her when she had few other options available, so she knew the value of reading better than most people ever will. Finally she chose to share her story not because she saw her starvation years as something heroic but because—like her parents before her and the husband she came to share her life with—she was civic minded. Elizabeth wanted to be useful, in her life and in her legacy. She had kept the story of her diabetes firmly behind closed doors, but she had no desire to control it after her death. We are all enriched by her generosity.

ABOUT THIS BOOK

I DO NOT HAVE diabetes, yet it has been an important element in my life. My father, Bill Thomson, had what was known in my childhood as juvenile diabetes, now called type 1 diabetes or insulin-dependent diabetes mellitus. I grew up easily able to cope with an occasional insulin reaction, and my mother kept the household to a strict mealtime routine to accommodate his condition. As a teenager, when I changed schools, type 1 diabetes was a point of connection between me and a new friend, Roz, whose father, Mick Rowe, had the disease, as did the mother of my friend Holly, who I met some years later. It was an important common thread in these friendships and it continued to be part of my life. My now ex-husband is a type 1 diabetic, as is one of my nieces. As the years passed, my expanding social circle included several diabetics and their families. While I can never really know what it is like to have this chronic illness, I have long been aware of the difficulties of living with it.

I knew nothing at all about what had happened to diabetics before insulin was discovered in 1922, so I was delighted to come across Michael Bliss's acclaimed book *The Discovery of*

Insulin. It was in those pages that I first met Elizabeth Evans Hughes. Bliss introduced her briefly to his readers as an example of a child who suffered from what was known in the early 20th century as simply "acute" diabetes as he told the great story of the research and the scientists involved. He was clearly engaged by this girl he called a "little Spartan," who lived for years on a starvation diet as a way of staving off death.

I was intrigued by Elizabeth and immediately made plans to travel from California to the Thomas Fisher Rare Book Library at the University of Toronto, where her letters from this period are part of "The Discovery of Insulin" collection. There, I immersed myself in her world and let her tell me her story. I found the "little Spartan" but, as I read, new questions arose. Where had this self-discipline come from? After all, few people of any age have this kind of self-control. What role did her family and early childhood play in instilling this quality? And most importantly, what sustained her? Even the Spartans had their gods and a whole social network to underpin and enforce their disciplined conduct. Where did Elizabeth's strength come from? What or who compelled or cajoled her? As I read and reread her letters, gathered information about her famous, politically powerful parents, her family, and her upbringing, and read widely on the period in which she had this crisis and on the experiences of the sick in general and sick children in particular, I slowly pieced together her emotional and social worlds.

Diabetes and indeed many other chronic illnesses are essentially isolating. But Elizabeth did not shut herself off. She tried her best in the face of enormous odds to live richly, filling her days with intellectual and social interests. She never lost hope that she was a girl with a future. She made every effort to stay connected to her family and friends, planning activities with them for months and years ahead.

Elizabeth Evans Hughes became, to paraphrase the words of Charles Dickens's David Copperfield, the hero of her own life. I hope you enjoy getting to know her and her journey as much as I did.

MANY PEOPLE HAVE helped me with this project. The diabetics in my social circle have been generous in talking to me about their experiences living with the disease. The librarians at the Thomas Fisher Rare Book Library, especially Jennifer Toews, have been welcoming and helpful, as have those at the Miner Library of the University of Rochester, the Library of Congress, and the Bermuda National Library, and Lisa Bayne at the Eli Lilly and Company Archives. I am grateful to Elizabeth Hughes's descendants, who have been generous with their time and their memories of their mother, and graciously allowed me access to her diaries and photographs from her later life. My thanks also go to Marion Gillespie for providing a home away from home on my trips to Toronto and to the University of the Pacific, for funding some of the travel for this project. I also greatly appreciate the research assistance of my students, Heather Mellon and Jeanette Sandoval.

Over the period I have been working on this book, a number of people have commented on the manuscript in its various forms and have shared many hours of conversation about it. Robert Middlekauff, as always, offered his gentle guidance. Gretchen Krueger, Diane Hill, Roz Gammie, Holly Levison, Merrill Schleier, Elly Sinacore, the late Jay Wessoff, Lisa Wrischnik, and Rebecca Davis all had thoughtful advice. Lisa Adams of Garamond Agency provided wise direction. My colleague Amy Smith read the whole manuscript and has been a wonderful sounding board. And to Michelle Krowl—what can I say? In addition to being my friend, a wonderful historian, and a kind host for many visits to Washington, D.C., she is a font of knowledge about the history of that city. When I needed to get my bearings on the Hugheses' physical world, she suggested we do a Hughes walking tour of the city. Armed with photocopied pages of the city directories from the period, we set off exploring. This was friendship indeed! And finally my thanks to my husband, Victor Ninov, for his unfailing enthusiasm and support.

BIBLIOGRAPHY

THIS BOOK RESTS on the letters of Elizabeth Evans Hughes deposited in the "Discovery of Insulin Collection" at the Fisher Library of the University of Toronto. I have gained detailed information about her life from several other sources, including her essay "My Father the Chief Justice," published in the *Supreme Court Historical Society 1976 Yearbook,* which sheds light on her early childhood. Historian Michael Bliss conducted an interview with her shortly before her death in 1981 and his notes are in the Michael Bliss Papers, "Notes and Interviews for the Discovery of Insulin," also in the Fisher Library; Bliss's essay "A Sudden Reprieve Called Insulin" appeared in *Saturday Night,* January 1982. Another source is Sandra Campbell, "A Sweet Life," *The Bermudian,* July 2000: 23–28. Elizabeth Hughes's children have generously made available to me her diaries from 1925–1934 and several surviving letters to her from her father. These documents are privately held by them. I have also benefited greatly from private communications from them regarding their reminiscences about their mother.

Much about the Hughes family and its social world comes from the Charles Evans Hughes papers in the Library of

Congress, newspapers, magazines, census records, and city directories. The 1921–1922 diaries of Anna Hamlin are part of the Charles S. Hamlin Papers, Library of Congress. Marlo Pusey's two-volume, Pulitzer and Bancroft prize–winning biography, *Charles Evans Hughes* (New York: Macmillan Company, 1951), has been invaluable. These are augmented by writings by contemporaries of the Hughes family, including Ida M. Tarbell, "How About Hughes?" *The American Magazine* 65:5, 451–64; Archibald Butt, *Taft and Roosevelt: The Intimate Letters of Archie Butt, Military Aide* (New York: Doubleday, Doran & Company, 1930); and the Mabel Boardman Papers, Library of Congress. My thanks to historian Michelle Krowl for locating these Hughes connections. James M. Goode, in *Capital Losses: A Cultural History of Washington's Destroyed Buildings* (Washington, DC: Smithsonian Institution Press, 1979), helped me imagine the city.

For the discovery of insulin, I have drawn on the archival sources at the University of Toronto "Discovery of Insulin Collection," especially the papers of Frederick Banting, Charles Best, and James Bertram Collip; the William Feasby Papers, which contain transcripts of Best's responses to Feasby's questions for his unpublished biography, were also helpful. I have additionally used contemporary newspapers and Alison Li, *J. B. Collip and the Development of Medical Research in Canada: Extracts and Enterprise* (Montreal: McGill-Queens University Press, 2003). Most importantly, I have drawn on Michael Bliss's definitive works, *The Discovery of Insulin* (Chicago: University of Chicago Press, 1982) and *Banting: A Biography* (Toronto: McClelland & Stewart Limited, 1984). I greatly admire both books.

Information on Jim Havens comes from the Banting Papers and Jim's and his father's correspondence in Letters of James S. Havens, Edward G. Miner Library, University of Rochester Medical Center, Rochester, New York; and Ralph Madeb, Leonidas Koniaris, and Seymour Schwartz, "The Discovery of Insulin: The Rochester, New York, Connection," *Annals of Internal Medicine* 143:12 (December 20, 2005), 907–12.

The scientific literature on diabetes in this era was extensive. Specifically, I drew on Lydia M. DeWitt, "Morphology and Physiology of Areas of Langerhans in Some Vertebrates," *Journal of Experimental Medicine* 8 (1906): 193–239; Frederick Allen, *Studies Concerning Glycosuria and Diabetes* (Cambridge, MA: Harvard University Press, 1913) and *Total Dietary Regulation in the Treatment of Diabetes* (New York: Rockefeller Institute, 1919); Elliott Joslin, *The Treatment of Diabetes Mellitus* (Philadelphia: Lea & Febiger, 1916) and *A Diabetic Manual for the Mutual Use of Doctor and Patient* (Philadelphia: Lea & Febiger, 1918); Moses Barron, "The Relation of Islets of Langerhans to Diabetes with Special Reference to Cases of Pancreatic Lithiasis," *Surgery, Gynecology & Obstetrics* 31 (1920): 437–48; and Israel Kleiner, "The Action of Intravenous Injections of Pancreatic Emulsions in Experimental Diabetes," *Journal of Biological Chemistry* 40 (1919): 153–70. Details of the impact of insulin on the first recipients can be found in Banting et al., "The Effects Produced on Diabetes by Extracts of Pancreas," *Transactions of the Association of American Physicians* (1922): 337–47; John Williams, "A Clinical Study of the Effects of Insulin in Severe Diabetes," *Journal of Metabolic Research* 2 (1922): 729–51; and H. Rawle Geyelin, George Harrop, Marjorie Murray, and Eugenia

Corwin, "The Use of Insulin in Juvenile Diabetes," *Journal of Metabolic Research* 2 (1922): 767–91. O. H. Gaebler, "Letter to the Editor," *Bulletin of the Canadian Biochemical Society* 2:3 (September 1965), 1, contains Gaebler's account of Collip identifying an insulin reaction for the first time. F. B. Michelson, "Rescued by Insulin," *Hygeia* 6 (1928): 672–75, showed that insulin still needed some promotion several years after the discovery.

Data on sickness and mortality come from Edwin A. M. Gale, "Perspectives in Diabetes: The Rise of Childhood Type 1 Diabetes in the 20th Century," *Diabetes* 51 (2002), 3353–61; "CDC on Infant and Maternal Mortality in the United States: 1900–99," *Population and Development Review* 25:4 (December 1999): 821–26; "CDC on Infectious Diseases in the United States, 1900-99," *Population and Development Review* 25:3 (September 1999): 635–40; Richard A. Meckel, "Levels and Trends of Death and Disease in Childhood, 1620 to the Present," *Children and Youth in Sickness and in Health: A Historical Handbook and Guide,* edited by Janet Golden, Richard A. Meckel, and Heather Munro Prescott (Westport, CT: Greenwood Press, 2004), pp. 3–24; and Richard C. Adelman and Lois M. Verbrugge, "Death Makes News: The Social Impact of Disease on Newspaper Coverage," *Journal of Health and Social Behavior* 41 (2000): 341–67.

There is a rich scholarship on the great medical scourges of this era, including James Flexner, *An American Saga: The Story of Helen Thomas and Simon Flexner* (Boston: Little Brown, 1984); John M. Barry, *The Great Influenza: The Epic Story of the Deadliest Plague in History* (New York: Viking Press, 2004); Anthony M. Lowell, *Tuberculosis: Tuberculosis Morbidity and*

Mortality and Its Control (Cambridge, MA: Harvard University Press, 1969); and Katherine Ott, *Fevered Lives: Tuberculosis in American Culture Since 1870* (Cambridge, MA: Harvard University Press, 1996). J. T. H. Connor, in *Doing Good: The Life of Toronto's General Hospital Toronto* (University of Toronto Press, 2000), shows how a research university and a large hospital responded to the challenges.

For information about the psychology of dying and chronically ill children, I have drawn on Myra Bluebond-Langner, *The Private Worlds of Dying Children* (Princeton, NJ: Princeton University Press, 1978); Cindy Dell Clark, *In Sickness and in Play: Children Coping With Chronic Illness* (New Brunswick, NJ: Rutgers University Press, 2003); and Chris Feudtner, *Bittersweet: Diabetes, Insulin, and the Transformation of Illness* (Chapel Hill: University of North Carolina Press, 2003). My thanks also to Dr. Feudtner, who is the Director of Research and Attending Physician, Palliative Care Team, Children's Hospital of Philadelphia, for his thoughts on Elizabeth Hughes shared in a private communication. Ross M. Hays, Geraldine Haynes, J. Russell Geyer, and Chris Feudtner, "Communication at the End of Life," *Palliative Care for Infants, Children, and Adolescents,* edited by Brian S. Carter and Marcia Levetown (Baltimore: Johns Hopkins University Press, 2004), pp. 112–40, also informed my thinking on this subject.

For the scholarship on letter writing, see David Barton and Nigel Hall, eds., *Letter Writing as Social Practice* (Philadelphia: John Benjamins Publishing Company, 2000).

For the way people write about illness, see Arthur Frank, *At the Will of the Body* (Boston: Houghton Mifflin, 1991); Arthur

Kleinman, *The Illness Narrative: Suffering Healing and the Human Condition* (New York: Basic Books, 1988); and G. Thomas Couser, *Recovering Bodies: Illness, Disability, and Life Writing* (Madison: University of Wisconsin Press, 1997).

To understand how Elizabeth may have perceived her body, I consulted Joan Jacobs Brumberg, *Fasting Girls: A History of Anorexia Nervosa* (New York: Vintage Books, 2000); Caroline Walker Bynum, *Holy Feast and Holy Fast: The Religious Significance of Food to Medieval Women* (Berkeley: University of California Press, 1987); Susan Bordo, *Unbearable Weight: Feminism, Western Culture and the Body* (Berkeley: University of California Press, 1993); and Laura Lovett, "The Popeye Principle: Selling Child Health in the First Nutritional Crisis," *Journal of Health Politics, Policy and Law* 30 (2005): 803–38. My thanks to Laura Lovett for some fruitful discussions.

On factors determining the onset of puberty, see Rose E. Frisch, "Fatness, Puberty, and Fertility: The Effects of Nutrition and Physical Training on Menarche and Ovulation," *Girls at Puberty: Biological and Psychosocial Perspectives,* edited by Jeanne Brooks-Gunn and Anne C. Petersen (New York: Plenum Press, 1983), pp. 29–49; and Julia A. Graber, Jeanne Brooks-Gunn, and Michelle P. Warren, "The Antecedents of Menarcheal Age: Heredity, Family Environment and Stressful Life Events," *Child Development* 66 (1995): 346–59.

There is an extensive literature on the larger meaning of children's books. I found the following especially helpful: Stephen Mintz, *Huck's Raft: A History of American Childhood* (Cambridge, MA: Belknap Press, 2004); Paula Fass and Mary Ann Mason, eds., *Childhood in America* (New York: New

York University Press, 2000); Gillian Avery, *Behold the Child: American Children and Their Books* (Baltimore: Johns Hopkins University Press, 1994); Heather Munro Prescott, "Stories of Childhood Health and Disease," *Children and Youth in Sickness and in Health,* edited by Janet Golden, Richard A. Meckel, and Heather Munro Prescott (Westport, CT: Greenwood Press, 2004), pp. 25–42; and John T. Dizer, Jr., *Tom Swift, The Bobbsey Twins, and Other Heroes of American Juvenile Literature* (Lewiston, ME: Edwin Mellen Press, 1997).

On the solace of beauty, Viktor M. Frankl, *Man's Search for Meaning: From Death-Camp to Existentialism,* translated by Gordon W. Allport (Boston: Beacon Press, 1962), provides a perspective that transcends place and time. The source of the quote from John Muir is *Our Nation's Parks* (New York: Houghton Mifflin, 1901). For the beauty of Bermuda especially, see Helen A. Cooper, *Winslow Homer Watercolors* (New Haven, CT: Yale University Press, 1986), on Homer's art. *Vogue,* January 15, 1921, and *National Geographic Magazine,* January 1922, contain the essays Elizabeth may have read near her departure date.

The background of Elizabeth's musical world comes from Laura Kuhn, ed., *Baker's Dictionary of Opera* (New York: Schirmer Books, 2000); "Parlor Songs: Popular Sheet Music from the 1800s to the 1920s," *www.parlorsongs.com/catalog/;* Barbara B. Heyman, *Barber: The Composer and His Music* (New York: Oxford University Press, 1994); and Timothy J. McGee, *The Music of Canada* (New York: W. W. Norton, 1985).

The special problems of being a political spouse are examined in Joyce Schuck, *Political Wives, Veiled Lives* (New York: Madison Books, 1991); and Katie Hickman, *Daughters of*

Britannia: The Lives and Times of Diplomatic Wives (New York: William Morrow, 1999).

For additional sources on the post-insulin world, Alfred R. Henderson, "Frederick M. Allen M.D., and the Psychiatric Institute at Morristown N.J. (1920–1938)," *Bulletin—Academy of Medicine of New Jersey* 16:4 (December 1940): 40–49, provided the rest of Allen's story. August Krogh's letter concerning the Nobel prize can be found in Jan Lindsten, "August Krogh and the Nobel Prize to Banting and Macleod," April 2, 2001, *www. nobelprize.org/nobel_prizes/medicine/articles/lindsten/.*

Illustrations on page 19 of the discoverers are from the Thomas Fisher Rare Book Library, University of Toronto as follows: Bert Collip, Collip Papers; Charles Best, Feasby Papers; Frederick Banting, Banting Papers; John Macleod, Best Papers. The images related to Elizabeth Hughes are as follows: Elizabeth with her mother on page 2, the Hughes family photograph on page 35, and Elizabeth's letter are from the Elizabeth Evans Hughes Papers, the Thomas Fisher Rare Book Library, University of Toronto; her diet records are from Banting Papers, the Thomas Fisher Rare Book Library, University of Toronto; and the image of the Hughes-Gossett family was made available by them. The photograph on page 204 of Elizabeth Hughes playing tennis is from the Library of Congress. The invitation to the Hugheses' Washington Conference reception is in the Anna Hamlin Scrapbook, Charles Hamlin Papers, Library of Congress. The cover of *St. Nicholas* magazine on page 137 is from the Library of Congress. The images of the boy identified only as J.L. on page 170 were kindly made available by Eli Lilly and Company Archives; and that of the unknown emaciated girl on page 55 appeared in H. Rawle Geyelin, George Harrop, Marjorie Murray, and Eugenia Corwin, "The Use of Insulin in Juvenile Diabetes," *Journal of Metabolic Research* 2 (1922): 767–91 and has been made available by the Thomas Fisher Rare Book Library, University of Toronto.

INDEX

145–49; team rediscovers insulin, 151–56; applying for patent, 155; and Jim Havens, 169; and other early recipients, 170; beginning clinical trials, 177–78; and Elizabeth Hughes, 179–81; life transformed by fame, 192–94; encourages Elizabeth to inject herself, 197–98; corresponds with Elizabeth, 204–05; Nobel Prize, 210–15, post-insulin career and death, 222–24

Banting, Henrietta B., 213

Banting Medal, 215

Barber, Samuel, 67–68

Barnard College, 209, 217, 223, 226

Barron, Moses, 46

Barrymore, Mrs. John, 89

Bermuda Trade Development Board, 128, 163,

Best, Charles, 18, 119, 151; background and military service, 20–21; an undergraduate at University of Toronto, 38; Banting's research assistant, 71–75; death of dogs, 73; observes Banting arguing with Macleod, 77–78; participates in new experiments, 92–95; American Physiological Society meeting, 117; restrains Banting, 119; cajoles Banting back to work, 145–49; applies for patent, 155; liked by Elizabeth Hughes, 192; given share in Nobel Prize, 210, post-insulin career and death, 213–14; comments on Elliott Joslin, 216

Best, Margaret M., 38, 74, 213

Beveridge, Wallace, 5

Black, Norman Irving, 134–35

Bliss, Michael, 224

Boardman, Mabel, 80, 206

Booth, Evangeline, 64–65

Booth, William, 64

Boston Symphony Orchestra, 189

Bradford, Gamaliel, 64

Brearley School, 23, 165,

Brown University, 24, 26, 31

Burgess, Blanche, xiv, 63, 66, 68, 79, 87, 90, 113, 150, 184, 188, 191, 193, 208, 224; on death and dying, 12; watchful of Elizabeth, 18, 56, 58; traveling to Glens Falls, 53–54; packing to leave, 76; traveling to Bermuda, 91–92, 95–97; remedy for seasickness, 92, 127; teamwork with Elizabeth, 103–04; writing, 109; and rowing, 120; Elizabeth's fall, 129; and reading, 145; news of insulin, 156–57; Catherine's wedding, 158; and enjoying flowers, 162; passing on gossip, 165–66; packing, 168; returning from Bermuda, 173; traveling to Toronto, 180–81; injecting insulin, 185; falling in love, 197; returning to Washington, 199; leaving, 202–03

Burnett, Frances Hodgson, 140, 190

Burroughs, John, 66

Butler, Alban, 61

C

Calvé, Emma, 189

Canadian Medical Association, 212

Carnegie, Andrew, 190

Carter, Wallace, 25–26

Chambers, Mrs., 184

246

Index